'If you want to increase your chance of conceiving a healthy baby, give yourself the strength to stay in treatment and improve your quality of life as you do so, it is vital for you to learn specific skills and strategies. In this book Ann Bracken has compiled what you need to know in an easily accessible, friendly and compassionate format.'

**Dr Alice D Domar, Associate Professor in Obstetrics, Gynaecology and Reproductive Biology, Harvard Medical School and Executive Director of the Domar Center for Mind/Body Health.**

'All too often the management of reproductive health is seen through the narrow prism of a particular clinician or clinic. This book provides the perfect balance outlining the integrative mind and body approach and provides an essential complement to the medical aspects of the fertility journey.'

**Dr James Nicopoullos, Consultant Gynaecologist and Sub-specialist in Reproductive Medicine, The Lister Hospital, Chelsea, London.**

'Ann Bracken expertly shows readers how to weave mindfulness into their lives to help them take care of their well-being as they live through a challenging process. Her book includes a great deal else besides, but I was impressed by how she makes mind-fulness so readily accessible.'

**Padraig O'Morain, Mindfulness teacher and Psychotherapist, author of *Mindfulness on the Go, Mindfulness for Worriers* and *Light Mind*.**

## ABOUT THE AUTHOR AND CONTRIBUTORS

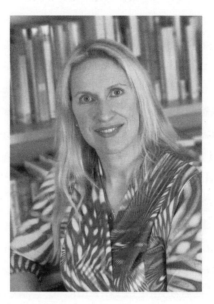

**Ann Bracken** is a leading protagonist in the area of Fertility Counselling. Her innovative and research-led work integrates mindfulness, psychotherapy and mind/body practices to support couples and individuals as they journey through the challenges and joys of natural and assisted fertility. A highly qualified and experienced Cognitive Behavioural Psychotherapist, Mindfulness Trainer and workshop facilitator, Ann has private counselling practices in Dublin, Ireland and Kensington, London. She also provides international consultations through her online counselling service www.fertilitycounsellingonline.com. A lecturer in the Department of Psychology at Glyndŵr University, Ann is also a part-time Senior Fertility Counsellor at the world-renowned

Lister Fertility Clinic, part of The Lister Hospital, Chelsea. As a certified Fertility Mind Body Programme trainer, Ann writes, delivers and facilitates fertility-specific workshops and training programmes for both clients and practitioners. Ann regularly writes feature articles and contributes to television and radio programmes on emotional and psychological health and well-being.

**Dr Alice D Domar, PhD** is the Executive Director of the Domar Center for Mind/Body Health, the Director of Integrative Care at Boston IVF and an Associate Professor, part-time, in Obstetrics, Gynaecology and Reproductive Biology at Harvard Medical School. She is a practising psychologist and researcher. Dr Domar is also on the board of directors for Resolve, the National Infertility Association in the US, and is the author or co-author of six books, including *Conquering Infertility*. She is the founder of the Mind/Body Program for Infertility and the author or co-author of more than 70 research articles, as well as the series editor of the books on the mind/body connection for Harvard Medical Publications. She travels internationally to speak on the relationship between stress and infertility. Her seventh book is *The Stress Bump* (2016). Further details can be found at www.domarcenter.com.

**Dr Marilyn Glenville, PhD** is one of the UK's leading nutritionists specialising in women's health. She is the former President of the Food and Health Forum at the Royal Society of Medicine. Dr Glenville obtained her doctorate from Cambridge University and regularly delivers at academic conferences. For over 30 years Dr Glenville has studied and practised nutrition, specialising in the natural approach to female hormone problems. She is a

# MIND BODY BABY

·······

## How to Overcome Stress and Enhance your Fertility with CBT, Mindfulness and Good Nutrition

### ANN BRACKEN

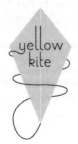

First published in Great Britain in 2016 by Yellow Kite
An imprint of Hodder & Stoughton
An Hachette UK company

1

Trade Paperback ISBN 978 1 473 62040 7
eBook ISBN 978 1 473 62041 4

Printed and bound by CPI Group (UK) Ltd, CR0 4YY

Hodder & Stoughton policy is to use papers that are natural, renewable and recyclable products and made from wood grown in sustainable forests. The logging and manufacturing processes are expected to conform to the environmental regulations of the country of origin.

*To my beautiful friend Mago – for your courage,*
*your heart and our shared laughter together*

# CONTENTS

# ACKNOWLEDGEMENTS

There are many significant people who encouraged and supported me in the writing of this book and in my passion for taking a Mind Body approach to fertility health and well-being.

Immense gratitude is owed to mindfulness author and Psychotherapist Padraig O'Morain for his encouragement and also his introduction to a wonderful agent, Susan Feldstein. Susan has supported me in such a positive way throughout. I also wish to acknowledge with immense gratitude Dr David Walsh and Mr Steve McGettigan of Sims IVF for encouraging and facilitating research undertaken to inform this book and for supporting my growth in the area of Fertility Mind Body health. I was fortunate as part of this to have gained from the wisdom and inspiration of Dr Alice Domar, Associate Professor of Obstetrics, Gynaecology and Reproductive Biology at Harvard Medical School, author in the field of Mind Body health and pioneer of Mind Body approaches to fertility. Her work continues to be an inspiration to me.

I have had a professional relationship with women's health expert and author Dr Marilyn Glenville for 15 years now and I am delighted that she contributed such an excellent chapter, highlighting the beneficial aspects of nutrition and supplements for fertility. I also want to acknowledge the generosity of Dr James Nicopoullos, Consultant Gynaecologist at The Lister Clinic in The Lister Hospital, Chelsea, for providing me with such interesting points for discussion and for his valuable help with the chapter on medical treatment. Respect and thanks go to John Hickey, an extraordinary supervisor, colleague and wonderful guide in self- and professional care in this interesting work we do.

I would also like to sincerely thank my family and friends, especially Sinead, Leighann, Joshua, Rhys and Isaac for ensuring that I still went out to play, a very important part of self-nurture even for writers, and, of course, thanks to Anthony for his unconditional love and those endless cups of tea! I would also like to thank Liza for her words of wisdom during this book's inception.

I would like to acknowledge the ongoing encouragement and insightful editorial input from Julia Kellaway, responsible for the editing of this book. In addition, much appreciation is extended to the overall editor, Liz Gough at Yellow Kite, for her valuable input throughout and believing wholeheartedly in the merits of its publication.

Importantly, I would like to thank all the women and men who have shared their hopes, vulnerabilities and healing with me and whom I have had the privilege of accompanying on their fertility journeys.

Humans have been asking themselves for years – what comes first, the chicken or the egg? And reproductive healthcare professionals have been asking a similar question for decades – does infertility cause stress or does stress cause infertility?

I consider myself to be a relatively intelligent, well-educated person and have been researching the stress/infertility question for almost 30 years, but the answer has just occurred to me. The answer to both questions is: why does it matter? Who cares? Why do we need to know if the chicken came first? Is it going to impact your enjoyment of scrambled eggs or roast chicken? I think not. For women and couples struggling with infertility who wonder about the impact of stress, is the direction of the causation vital information?

My answer is no. If you accept the premise that infertility causes stress, that should be motive enough to do something about it. As a psychologist, my main goal is to decrease emotional suffering. I have always said that pregnancy is a delightful side effect in women who have learned new stress-management skills. The main focus should be on improving the quality of life of our patients. If they subsequently get pregnant, that is truly awesome.

But if they don't get pregnant, it is vital that each one has the coping skills and support to keep herself emotionally healthy.

Infertility is stressful. There is data which shows that women who are experiencing infertility have equivalent levels of anxiety and depression to women with cancer, heart disease and HIV+ status. Procreation is a strong instinct and thus being denied the possibility of becoming pregnant and having a baby can cause severe distress. That is a normal reaction to infertility. It is entirely normal to feel badly about one's body, to struggle to communicate with your partner, to want to avoid siblings and friends who conceive easily, to resent the time that infertility takes away from your job, to worry about the cost of treatment, and even to wonder why God isn't answering your prayers to have a healthy baby. It can impact every area of your life, and yet well-meaning family and friends tend to make suggestions and comments which suggest it's your fault: 'Just relax', 'You're trying too hard', 'Just adopt', 'Go on vacation.' Each comment implies that if you would simply do something differently, you would conceive. So if you find yourself feeling anxious, sad, irritable or lonely, it means one thing: you are having an entirely normal reaction to infertility. Staying emotionally healthy during infertility can be a true challenge.

This also means that you need to pay attention to the data which suggests that stress might contribute to infertility. Women who are highly stressed take longer to get pregnant and some research shows that women who are the most depressed and/or anxious also may have lower pregnancy rates from IVF. But here is the where the chicken/egg question arises. Women who know they have a good prognosis before starting a cycle are likely to be less anxious and sad. So if they get pregnant, is it because they were less stressed or because they were a good candidate for IVF?

Women who know they have a poor prognosis before starting a cycle are far more likely to feel really worried about the outcome. So if they don't get pregnant, was it because of their stress or because of egg quality? We can't tease apart these factors. What we do know, however, is that women who are struggling with infertility who learn coping skills, specifically relaxation and stress management, do have higher pregnancy rates. We don't know exactly why – I personally don't care; as long as it works, why worry about why it works? – but the most recent research shows that women who learn how to decrease their stress levels have significantly higher pregnancy rates and lower levels of psychological symptoms than women who don't learn these techniques.

Which brings me to the reason for writing this foreword: to introduce you to *Mind Body Baby*. If you want to increase your chance of conceiving a healthy baby, give yourself the strength to stay in treatment and improve your quality of life as you do so, it is vital for you to learn specific skills and strategies. In this book Ann Bracken has compiled what you need to know in an easily accessible, friendly and compassionate format.

I have treated thousands of individuals and couples who are experiencing infertility. I know all too well how challenging a process it can be. I also know how hard it can be to take care of yourself, especially during times of crisis. But in this case, it is absolutely necessary. If you care about your emotional health in addition to your physical health, keep on reading . . .

**Dr Alice D Domar, Associate Professor in Obstetrics, Gynaecology and Reproductive Biology, Harvard Medical School and Executive Director of the Domar Center for Mind/Body Health**

# Taking an Integrative Approach to Your Fertility Health

..................................................

I have spread my dreams under your feet;
Tread softly because you tread on my dreams.

WB YEATS

..................................................

Hospital visits, calendar watching, ongoing test results and scheduled sex can make trying for a baby a stressful experience, and the strain it puts on couples and individuals struggling with fertility problems can impact hugely. With an approach that puts well-being at the heart of fertility, *Mind Body Baby* offers a proven successful alternative to formal counselling, providing help and guidance on how to enhance and improve your outcome.

As a Fertility Counsellor and Cognitive Behavioural Psychotherapist, I have worked with many individuals and couples over the years, and have seen the proven benefits for those who invest in their psychological, emotional and physical health on their fertility journey. *Mind Body Baby* explains how to integrate evidence-based psychological and physical treatment approaches to enhance fertility using medical and natural health-care. For some readers, this will involve taking a natural healthcare approach, while others will need to seek assisted reproductive care, and many will benefit from a combination of both. By committing to taking an integrative approach to your health, you are embracing an active role in your fertility care and well-being for mind and body.

This book is specifically written with fertility in mind and incorporates mindfulness-based stress reduction for fertility, cognitive behavioural therapy (CBT), nutrition, relationship enhancing skills and journaling to heal. It also pays attention to your physical health and stress reduction by including restorative yoga and mindful movement with complementary health and lifestyle guidance. Women's health expert, Dr Marilyn Glenville, contributes an excellent chapter on how to boost fertility with nutrition, a pre-conception plan and supplements. Each chapter also includes skills to reduce stress and optimize your fertility journey – whether natural or assisted.

*Mind Body Baby* includes a practical guide to assisted reproductive treatment options, who they are recommended for and their implications, as well as the latest research regarding the relationship between fertility and stress. This chapter contains everything you need to know to engage with your consultant and fertility choices in an informed and empowered way, putting you and your partner at the centre of your treatment process.

It is natural when you are facing fertility problems that you experience emotional symptoms that can feel overwhelming and difficult to manage. The exercises on mindful awareness will increase your ability to be aware and present to difficult feelings or sensations without being pulled out of your emotional centre, while the mindfulness-based stress reduction techniques have been scientifically proven to help overcome the stress and anxiety associated with fertility problems. The section on CBT will support you to positively change negative fertility thoughts to more self-accepting and compassionate ones. Mindfulness and CBT are proven therapeutic approaches that help individuals to manage stress-inducing conditions and overcome feelings of low mood or anxiety. It makes sense that a healthy mind benefits your body and a healthy body benefits your mind. Each chapter will provide helpful tools to enable you to improve your mind and body health and to support your fertility in a hands-on and effective way.

Managing fertility issues affects your mind, body and relationships and so ensuring that you take care of these areas maximizes your experience. Whether you need some reflective and decision-making time with journaling before deciding on a treatment approach, or you need to bring more intimacy and loving feelings back into your relationship, *Mind Body Baby* will show you how to invest in yourself and each other in addition to your treatment. The book aims to help you and your partner more easily manage the challenges relating to fertility and improve your mind–body health and relationship connections. Ultimately it is my hope that you will become a kind and generous friend to yourself and each other and not get lost in the fertility process.

*Mind Body Baby* provides you with step-by-step guidance to focus on optimizing your chances of conception by gaining the insights needed to help you choose and integrate the best natural and medical treatment approaches available. The practical information and guidance in this book will help you to make confident choices and effectively navigate your fertility journey in a way that is right for you, individually and as a couple. May you travel well.

# CHAPTER 1

# Managing the Psychological and Emotional Impact of Fertility Problems

..........................................

Hope is a waking dream.

ARISTOTLE

..........................................

It is estimated that 72.4 million women globally experience fertility problems[1] and their impact is far-reaching. Fertility problems impinge on an individual's physical health and their relationships with others while also adding pressure on work and social situations. Infertility is classified as an inability to conceive after 12 months of unprotected sexual intercourse. For some couples, it may mean achieving a successful pregnancy but experiencing repeated miscarriage, while for others their experience of infertility is 'secondary infertility' – where they have had a child in the past but are unable to conceive a subsequent child. Infertility problems affect 1 in 6 couples worldwide,[2] although for the individual and couple coping with infertility problems, it can feel like an isolating and lonely experience.

It is generally recommended that couples seek help via their GP after 12 months of trying to conceive. However, if the woman is over 35, they should visit their GP after six months of trying without success, as there may be many contributing factors that need assessment.

It is difficult to gain perspective in a world filled with temperature gauging, possible injections and timed sexual intercourse. A client I worked with recently likened it to being like Alice in Alice and Wonderland except that, in her situation, she had fallen down a hole into the world of infertility where nobody understood how she felt or what she was going through, and that this world became bigger and bigger to eventually take over her universe. Learning to come back out of the hole and deal with fertility problems as part of life helps to manage this difficult situation in a more harmonious way and to bring intuitive wisdom back to your decision-making.

In 2013, I undertook research[3] with 228 fertility patients using the fertility quality of life measurement tool FertiQoL. This tool was developed over eight years by the American Society for Reproductive Medicine (ASRM) and the European Society of Human Reproduction and Embryology (ESHRE) in collaboration with Cardiff University[4] and the biopharmaceutical company Merck Serono. It assesses the impact of infertility issues across important areas, such as 'general health, self perceptions, emotions, partnership, family and social relationships, work life and future life plans'.[5] The areas impacted most negatively by experiencing fertility problems included self-esteem, emotions, social situations and future life plans. The participants reported the following:

- 57 per cent expressed that their attention and concentration were impaired by thoughts of infertility.

- 46 per cent described feeling 'completely' or 'to a great extent' 'drained or worn out because of fertility problems'.
- 83 per cent expressed that they fluctuate between hope and despair very often due to their fertility problems.
- 80 per cent stated that they experience symptoms of grief.

An interesting finding was that only 20 per cent of respondents sought counselling support for these significant issues. This may be because many women and men already feel somewhat stigmatized managing a fertility-related diagnosis and could perceive the need to seek fertility counselling as adding to this. However, perhaps seeing it as a situation in your life that will not last forever but may benefit from emotional and psychological support may help if you feel you need to seek it. The Royal College of Obstetricians and Gynaecologists stated that there are dangers of neglecting 'the emotional impact of involuntary childlessness and viewing it solely in biological or medical terms'.[6] They describe fertility counselling as an amalgam of medicine and medical health, outlining the importance of counselling for those affected by infertility.[7]

## Fertility Counselling or Psychotherapy

The aim of counselling or psychotherapy to support you on your fertility journey should ideally include the following:

- To support you in reclaiming your self-confidence and help you to feel more empowered when going through the fertility treatment process and beyond.

* To give you dedicated time and space to nurture and enhance your relationship with yourself and your partner.
* To learn effective coping skills, for example for the two-week wait and awaiting test results.
* To support you in decreasing or overcoming difficult feelings associated with fertility, for example stress, anxiety, jealousy, low mood or fatigue.
* To support your physical health – a healthy mind supports a healthy body. For example, depressed individuals find it more difficult to engage with health-promoting activities.
* To work with you on your expectations regarding treatment and treatment outcomes as you consider your options.
* To integrate skills aimed at increasing feelings of self-compassion and kindness.
* To explore the implications of certain treatments and discuss the gains and losses in the shorter and longer term before making your decisions.
* To help you with managing or overcoming psychosexual problems. Depending on the length of time and severity of the symptoms, this may require that you attend a psychosexual therapist.
* To support a healthy attitude towards your treatment choices. For example, a positive attitude towards disclosure regarding genetic origins with a child has been shown to correlate with increased positive interactions between mothers and their child born from egg donation.[8] It would be reasonable to assume that experiencing feelings of acceptance towards yourself, your partner and your

treatment decisions will increase positive feelings if you have a child from the process.

* To work on changing any unhelpful beliefs (either towards yourself or others) into more positive and helpful ones.
* To help you to manage the emotional impact of treatment.
* To help you to develop coping strategies for dealing with other people's pregnancies and also learn how to work with the reactions of families, friends or work colleagues.
* To help change unhelpful thinking styles into more self-accepting ones that support rather than hinder you through the process. Some thoughts actually maintain sadness, guilt, anxiety or low mood, for example, 'nothing good ever happens to us'.
* To provide psycho-educational material and lifestyle infor-mation support to enhance your experience during treatment and beyond.

There are many and diverse counselling and psychotherapeutic approaches and it will be more effective if you choose the coun-selling most appropriate to your needs. It is advisable to do some initial research into the counselling help you are looking for. Ensure that your counsellor or psychotherapist is qualified with professional accreditation and ask what particular counselling modality they work in. Recent legislation in the UK and Ireland has outlined that a counsellor/psychotherapist is registered on the government's register for professional standards to ensure that they meet sufficient educational and skills-based require-ments. To be registered in the US as a professional counsellor or psychotherapist, it is required that the mental health practitioner is trained to a minimum of Master's degree level with post-graduate experience. Ascertaining the level of training and experience undertaken by your therapist is a good first step in finding the right therapist for you. It is also important when working with fertility-related issues that your therapist has additional training and experience in this area.

Research provided by Professor Sarah Berga and presented at the European Society for Human Reproduction and Embryology conference stated that women who received CBT observed over 20 weeks experienced an increase in self-esteem. In addition, ovulation was restored in 80 per cent of the women, indicating that therapy can benefit women on a physical and psychological level. According to Professor Berga, 'behavioural and psychological interventions that address problematic behaviours and attitudes, such as CBT, have the potential to permit a resumption of full ovarian function along with recovery of the adrenal, thyroidal and other neuroendocrine aberrations'.[9]

Of course, fertility counselling or psychotherapy is one form of support. There are many other ways we can improve our emotional, psychological and physical health and well-being, as outlined in the chapters that follow.

## When Emotions Feel Overwhelming

Everybody navigates their fertility journey differently and this is also true within relationships. However, the stress associated with treatment can become very burdensome and self-care is paramount. In a study of 211 patients who had undertaken in-vitro fertilization, patients were asked why they had stopped treatment.[10] The most common reason given (as expressed by 41 per cent of participants) was the psychological burden and a need to have a break. Managing the psychological and emotional impact of treatment will ensure that you remain self-empowered and resilient, whatever your decision choices.

Helping yourself to manage the roller coaster of emotions begins with recognizing the presenting symptoms and when to seek self-help or professional support. While it is unrealistic to expect that any woman or man would not experience some distress relating to a diagnosis or treatment, it is worth understanding the difference between experiencing anxiety levels of stress and concerned levels of stress, or depression compared with sadness, as this can indicate when problems may be deepening.

## Anxiety versus Concern

| Anxiety | Concern |
| --- | --- |
| *Types of thinking:* | *Types of thinking:* |
| • Overestimates the level of threat and how things will work out: 'This absolutely won't work.' | • Is realistic about the issue at hand: 'This is difficult but it's worth it for what we want.' |
| • Underestimates ability to cope: 'I can't stand this.' | • Is realistic about abilities to manage: 'I can do this because I did it the last time.' |
| • Creates a bigger threat than the existing one: 'He will leave me if this doesn't work.' | • Does not create a bigger threat than is there: 'We will get through this together.' |
| • Finds it difficult to think clearly – has a racing mind. | • Can concentrate on other things with clarity of mind. |

*What you do because of your thinking and feelings:*

- Probably disengage from further treatment even if you are in a group of patients where it is deemed highly likely to succeed.
- Won't want to think or deal with anything to do with fertility.
- May begin to become super-stitious about how to deal with things. This can become costly!
- Avoid difficult feelings by numbing out with food, alcohol or other excessive activities, for example, overwork or shopping.
- May seek constant reassurance from others, for example, seeking many opinions for the same problem (visiting the doctor four or five times for each issue).

- Make wise choices about where, when and how much treatment to have.
- Face the fertility problem and choose the best course of action.
- Research and decide on what action to take to increase likelihood of success.
- Manage feelings and can continue being fully present with day-to-day experiences.

## Depression versus Sadness

| Depression | Sadness |
| --- | --- |

*Types of thinking:*

- Can only think and focus on the negative outcome and very little else.
- Thinks of it as a personal failure rather than as a failure of the treatment working.
- Begins to perceive themselves as completely helpless in this situation and perhaps in life in general.
- Connects it to all other losses experienced in the recent and distant past.
- Feels hopeless about the future.

- Allows thoughts and feelings of sadness with acceptance. Recognizes that this is a negative outcome and not of their making. Tends to gain some insights and moves forward with this new learning.
- Thinks of ways to take care of themselves and their partner.
- Thinks about the present and feels sad. However, can plan and think about the future with hope.

*What you do because of your thinking and feelings:*

- Withdraw from all reminders. This may mean totally withdrawing yourself from any fertility clinics or from friends who have children. This is not the same as a considered ending of treatment.
- Stop social and interactive activities for prolonged periods of time.

- May seek solace in your own company for a while, however will re-engage with supportive friends and family (not non-supportive ones during this time!).
- Will allow feelings of loss while also taking gentle care of yourself.

- Shuts down and relies on one's own company. Mistrusts others.
- Creates an environment that mirrors one's own beliefs – 'Nobody cares' – while also does not make contact with others or reply to those reaching out.
- May engage in self-sabotaging behaviours, for example end a relationship because of fear that their partner will leave if the treatment does not work.
- May remove themselves from many day-to-day activities.

- Will reach out to trustworthy friends or family to share and express your sense of loss.
- Will integrate self-care and healing in their process of recovery.
- Can engage with day-to-day activities although experiencing a sense of sadness.

---

Once you become aware of the times when you are thinking and feeling negatively, the good news is that you can begin to bring positive change to what you do or how you are thinking about yourself and the situation.

Cognitive behavioural therapy and mindfulness exercises encourage a deeper awareness of how you are thinking, how you are feeling and what you are doing to help or hinder your emotional progress. It is naturally important to allow yourself to experience your feelings. However, it is also helpful to gain support if you feel overwhelmed by them. The CBT thought records and positive self-statements in Chapter 7 (pages 178 and 179) will provide you with insights and alternatives to gain different perspectives and more self-compassion. If you find that these feelings are not alleviating, it may be time to seek therapeutic support with fertility counselling.

## Grief: A Special Kind of Loss

Grief associated with fertility can mean several things:

* the loss of a hoped-for child if a treatment hasn't worked;
* loss as you discover that a positive pregnancy test has actually been a 'chemical pregnancy'; or
* loss following a miscarriage in the early or late stages of pregnancy.

It is hard to deal with loss at any time. However, it can be even more challenging if you are holding feelings of grief while also planning another cycle of treatment. It can also be difficult to manage the stages of grief if those around you don't know about or appreciate your loss.

Recognizing the process of loss can sometimes help you to adjust to it and move through it as best you can. It is important to give expression to your feelings and also to integrate ways to support yourself to overcome rather than get stuck in them. In 1969, Elisabeth Kübler-Ross, a psychiatrist in Switzerland, outlined the stages of grief as being: shock, anger, bargaining, depression and acceptance.[11] These are often expanded upon to reflect different experiences of loss and shock – denial, bargaining, anger, low mood, testing and acceptance are feelings not uncommon to individuals and couples experiencing fertility-related loss. Naturally, not everybody will experience loss in the same way, even if they are individuals within the same relationship, overcoming the same loss. Equally, not everybody will experience all of these stages or in this order. However, dealing with fertility-related loss may mean that you and/or your partner could experience the following:

### Stage 1: Shock

It takes time to come to terms with loss, whether it is a negative outcome or overcoming the trauma of miscarriage. Initial feelings can include numbness and disbelief, followed by anxious thinking – 'I must do something now to change this' – and a feeling of being disorientated.

**Self-care:** It can really help to give yourself some time out from daily activities to dedicate time to self-care and nurture by being your own best friend during this time (See Chapter 8, page 189).

### Stage 2: Denial

Part of the denial process is a denial that this is real. It can bring up some very strong and challenging feelings including guilt, sadness and a deep yearning for your hoped-for baby, while you may also find it very difficult to be present to your feelings of loss. This can be accompanied by huge fear and you may find yourself with excess nervous energy and begin strategizing to establish a next-phase plan. Though planning is important, we don't always make our best decisions during this vulnerable phase.

**Express it:** Talking about how you feel may need to happen over and over before you feel that you are coming to terms with how things are in this moment. Expressing strong feelings of fear, regret, anger and frustration in a healthy way, for example focusing on the source of these strong feelings, allows you to process them without transferring them on to other people and situations around you.

### Stage 3: Bargaining

During this phase you may find yourself going over every detail of the treatment cycle or experience leading up to the loss. Often this is characterized by a real lack of self-kindness as you find small details and opportunities to berate yourself with, for example, 'I should have gone to this clinic over that one . . .', 'I should have started this sooner . . .', 'I should have noticed that I was not feeling too good earlier and visited the hospital for a check-up . . .'. This lack of self-kindness takes present information (not available at the time of the loss) and tries to apply it to the experience in the past in an effort to change the current situation. As you will note from the above, bargaining is often characterized by a personal overuse of internal 'shoulds', 'musts' and 'ought to haves'!

**Focus on the present:** Mindfulness-based practice will help you to focus on the present without judging yourself and allowing (although perhaps not liking) you to be in the now moments more, thus not trying to take on too much from the past, present and future. Although it is natural for past thoughts to rekindle present sadness, managing them so that you are not over-whelmed is kinder than chastising yourself through them. The grief in itself is enough to carry without adding self-blame. (See Chapter 2, page 22.)

### Stages 4 and 5: Anger and Depression (or Low Mood)

It is completely natural that feelings of loss bring up other strong feelings, such as anger, resulting from the frustrations of our life's aspirations being dashed. However, this anger can quickly develop into the blame game – either blaming yourself, your partner or the clinician you consulted. While it is very important to work out areas of beneficial change before moving forward, it is also important that you don't overattribute blame to yourself or another person in the frustration of trying to overcome loss. Equally, it is probably not the best time to chal-lenge another difficult person or situation you are currently dealing with!

For a time, low mood or depression may accompany the pain-ful feelings of not having what your heart yearns for most, and you may feel somewhat helpless in this process.

**Journaling:** Writing a letter (not an email!) to yourself, your partner or the clinician but not sending it can be a helpful way to express and process deep and difficult feelings and to move forward through them. Follow the self-healing journaling exer-cises in Chapter 2 (page 47-52) to help you understand and move through these difficult feelings. Eventually you can begin to make a plan to move forward that fits more easily, as you will have come to it naturally rather than feeling forced to come up with one.

## Stage 6: Testing

When overcoming fertility-related loss, the individual or couple may begin to consider their 'Plan B': now that this has happened, what next? This testing phase may include considering the gains and losses, in the short and long term, of many options. Although difficult, if you acknowledge and work through your feelings they are less likely to manifest in other areas of your life, for example, being passive-aggressive or blaming another because you feel sad or frustrated. Grieving takes its own time. The testing phase is a valid phase which can help you to move forward and find realistic and acceptable solutions to begin to work towards.

**Solution-focused problem-solving:** Outlining your personal needs and desires and how best to work towards them may require that you consider many options and the gains and losses in the short and long term for yourself and others. Chapter 3 can help you in reaching a decision as it outlines points to consider when undertaking medical treatment. You can also integrate some self-nurturing activities outlined in Chapter 8 to help with looking after yourself while in the decision-making process.

### Stage 7: Acceptance

Rebuilding your life after experiencing a loss involves gaining an acceptance of where you are now and how best to move forward. It involves accepting the loss and learning how to bring balance and positive feelings back into your life and towards yourself again. Although you may have a different perspective, you can begin to engage with your life again with hope and appreciation. During this phase individuals usually re-engage with social connections, for example, once again feeling connected to friends, their partner, family and co-workers.

**Journaling:** Take some time to connect with your strengths. If you cannot think of any, ask three friends to name one of your strengths or things they admire about you and trust in what they tell you!

Knowing and reconnecting with your strengths can help you to draw on them in the present and future. Strengths can include: open-mindedness, kindness, forgiveness, friendliness, resilience, being hard-working, good sense of humour, expressing gratitude, being motivated, persistent, brave, having an appreciation of beauty, etc. Write about your top three strengths and how these positive qualities help you when you experience difficulties. This exercise can help to increase feelings of life satisfaction and personal well-being.

## Other Difficult Feelings

Other common and difficult feelings experienced during this time can be jealousy or envy towards close friends. Women often express frustration at hearing that yet another friend has got pregnant so easily. Guilt can quickly follow on the heels of envy as you begin to feel like a really bad friend for feeling this way.

It is completely natural to be envious or frustrated when you are struggling and investing so much into the treatment for your hoped-for child. This is especially true if you perceive others as sailing through the experience. It can help to keep in mind that you are managing a medical problem and that, although this medical problem means you can still work and socialize, it is a physical problem that impacts on the reproductive area of your (or your partner's) body. Your friends do not have this medical problem, although they may have other life problems to deal with.

Show yourself some understanding during these challenging times. Perhaps instead of visiting your friend in hospital after she has had a baby, you could send flowers and a message wishing her the best – you will usually find once you explore your feelings a little deeper that you mean her no harm and do want the best for her, so this message is true. The feelings of envy are an acknowledgement of your own hurt and are passing in nature. Also, remember that you are doing your very best to have the same and this may be your reality very soon!

Chapter 7 will help you to reflect more fully on your thoughts and feelings and view your difficulties from different perspectives. Where necessary, you can learn to challenge any unhelpful thinking styles using the CBT thought records to map your thoughts, feelings and what you do (see pages 178–9). You can combine this with some self-nurturing and distracting activities along with mindfulness-based stress reduction outlined in the following chapter (page 40) to resource yourself fully on your fertility journey.

Having optimum psychological, physical and emotional health while managing a fertility health problem will at the very least support you to undertake treatment without being emotionally overwhelmed by it and, based on the research available, is likely to enhance your chances of conceiving while doing so.

# CHAPTER 2

## *Mindfulness Practice*

........................................................................

You can't stop the waves but you can learn to surf.
JON KABAT-ZINN, DIRECTOR OF MINDFULNESS
IN MEDICINE, HEALTHCARE AND SOCIETY,
UNIVERSITY OF MASSACHUSETTS

........................................................................

The emotional waves associated with facing fertility problems can feel overwhelming at times. Whether you are waiting to undertake a pregnancy test each month or anticipating test results and making decisions relating to treatment options, worrying thoughts about the future can often lead to feelings of anxiety and despair. Being faced with a range of options without certainty often leads to increased confusion and stress, and raises questions such as:

- Do we try a natural approach to enhance our fertility and, if so, for how long, or do we book an appointment for assisted reproductive treatment?
- Do we continue with intrauterine insemination or move on to in-vitro fertilization?

* Do we consider donor options or are we dealing with the end of treatment?

Mindfulness brings a more gentle awareness to the fertility process and increases your ability to be honest with yourself about what is present with you on a feeling, thinking and physical level as each fertility-related experience arises. Mindfulness enables you to become consciously present to an experience without being swept away by the feelings or thoughts we associate with it. Often our challenging experiences are deepened by the stories we tell ourselves about the situation.

This mindful awareness has been described as 'the awareness that emerges through paying attention on purpose, in the present moment, and non-judgementally to things as they are'.[1] The opposite to mindful awareness is having an automatic-pilot approach to living, for example, driving the car to and from the medical clinic without noticing any of the journey, or being hostile towards others without self-reflection or considering the impact of your actions. We often become busy overthinking and excessively doing – for example, excessive shopping, overworking or using technology to engage unnecessarily with social media – as a way of avoiding what we truly feel and to distract ourselves from our thoughts. While it is important to do this sometimes, it can become a habit where the virtual and doing world is more real than the actual lived experience in our environment (for example, when eating breakfast we don't taste or experience it as we're busy planning our lunch or the day ahead). This can quite easily happen in the fertility process as we travel back in our mental time machine to try and change details in the past, or travel in our future time machine to determine absolutes about when, where and how it should be. Having freedom from this way of thinking brings a deeper calm and consequently lowers our stress levels, even in challenging moments. Being in our moment-to-moment experience as much as possible is more energizing and stress-reducing as we're not managing fears relating to our past or perceived future.

Mindfulness is described as a 'practice' as it requires a commitment to engage with it, in its many forms, to truly benefit from it. This ancient practice can be traced back to Buddhist meditative approaches. However, aspects of stillness meditation have also been present in Christianity, Taoism, Judaism and Hinduism. Mindfulness has now become a universal secular practice and in recent years has been integrated into psychology, education, medicine, business and, perhaps most surprisingly, politics! *TIME* magazine recently referred to a 'Mindful Revolution' on their front cover and described the benefits of mindfulness as including 'finding peace in a stressed-out, digitally dependent culture'.[2]

The other benefits of mindfulness include an increased awareness of our sensory experiences and the ability to observe our habitual thought patterns. In so doing, we gain increased insight into our lived experiences, good and bad, and let go of unhelpful thinking and beliefs, which can often serve as a running commentary to everyday events. Research has shown that mindfulness significantly improves psychological and physical health and overall well-being.

By undertaking formal and informal mindfulness practices, we nurture our mind–body connection. Formal practices include taking time each day to focus our attention on our breath, body sensations, thoughts, feelings and senses in exercises that may include:

- sitting meditations (page 185)
- the three-minute mindful check-in (page 27)
- the body scan (page 57)
- walking meditations (page 161)
- body presence (for example, restorative yoga – see Chapter 6)
- loving-kindness meditations (page 205)

Informal practices include bringing moment-to-moment awareness to our daily activities; whether brushing our teeth or attending an appointment with a fertility consultant, we can aim to bring mindful awareness to that experience.

In the West, we are usually drawn to mindfulness because we need to change something in our lives, rather than it being part of our cultural experience. As such, we can also bring a lot of expectations that it must work! Part of the learning is to let go of these expectations and demands about how we 'should' be or what mindfulness 'should' do and adopt what is known as a 'beginner's mind'.[3] Ideally you will cultivate the following in your mindfulness practice:

- **Non-judgement:** being an impartial witness to your thoughts, emotions and physiological experiences that arise.
- **Patience:** allowing your mindful experience to deepen over time and practice.
- **A beginner's mind:** being receptive to the unfolding experience rather than blocking yourself with 'expert' analysis about how it shouldn't, couldn't or wouldn't work!

- **Trust:** trusting in the wisdom of your feelings and intuition, which allow you to reconnect with your authentic self, rather than seeking constant reassurance outside of yourself.

- **Non-striving:** letting go of the 'purpose' of meditation and just paying attention to your moment-to-moment experience. This allows you to be okay just as you are, in this moment, rather than being overly present to thoughts such as, 'Right, I will do this now for 15 minutes as I need to relax so this better work to help me to de-stress as I can't manage this stress!'.

- **Acceptance:** acceptance does not mean things won't change, as life is always changing. However, it allows you to let go of emotionally charged feelings of resistance, which in turn brings you more peace of mind and less physical tension. In mindfulness we are open to accepting ourselves in this present moment while also holding an understanding that we are experiencing fertility problems. (We have fertility problems, we are not a problem with fertility issues).

- **Letting go:** nurturing a mind of letting go or non-attachment supports you being present to where you are now, not drifting into past regrets or future worries. We 'let go' of thoughts, feelings or situations, whether pleasant or unpleasant, in our meditation. We notice the experience without attachment – an injection is an injection, as it is, rather than accompanied by additional negative internal dialogue about the injection. We notice that fear is present but do not engage with a negative story, for example, 'I hate this injection. I really could be doing without it. Why do I have to have it now?', and therefore over-focus on the sensation. Instead, we notice the feeling as a sensation and notice the thoughts as mental events passing through our mind. Thoughts are not facts.

## The Three-minute Mindful Check-in

Let's begin with a three-minute mindful check-in. Taking time to pause and focus on the present moment can help us to lean away from ruminating on if, when or how our pregnancy will be achieved. Though we continue to hold our positive, clear intention of having a pregnancy, we move towards the present moment more. On each out-breath we aim to let go of our striving, planning, sometimes critical self, and with each in-breath we begin to rest in a more accepting and kinder self where our true nature lies.

Find a quiet and comfortable environment; one where you are least likely to be disturbed and preferably without too much background noise or distraction.

- Sit in a comfortable position with your back reasonably upright. Allow your eyes to close and rest during the exercise.
- Take a few long, deep breaths:
  - breathing in; through your nose, all the way in, noticing that your stomach rises softly with each full in-breath;
  - breathing out; letting go on the out-breath, with your

mouth loosely shaped in a circle (as though to whistle), gently and without effort.

- Allow yourself to arrive more deeply into your body with each breath. As you breathe in you may wish to say the word 'calm' in your mind and, on your out-breath, the words 'letting go'.

- Notice what feelings are present for you now. Simply notice the emotional tone that is here with you in the moment. Feelings may be pleasant or unpleasant; just notice them and continue in your awareness of your in- and out-breaths.

- As you become more present to how you are feeling, you may also become aware of sensations in your body. Bring your attention to these sensations. Do you feel tense or relaxed? Simply notice that these are the sensations that you are carrying in your body now.

- Practise becoming aware and present with regards to your feelings, sensations and thoughts. Notice that thoughts come and go. There is no need to follow your thoughts and create stories; there is no need to work things out. Just become a 'witness' to your thoughts as they arrive, pass and leave. Spend some minutes just 'checking in' and simply allowing what is in your present experience to come to the fore.

It can be helpful to identify times when you could integrate your check-in within your normal day, for example, at the beginning of your lunch break; before the next board meeting; when you park your car in the driveway of the clinic; or before you enter the house. You can do the check-in several times during the day to re-centre yourself, even if the winds of change blow around you and your daily demands beckon.

**Keep a Mindfulness Fertility Log**

After your three-minute check-in, notice any changes when you resume your activities. Take some time to write about the thoughts, feelings and sensations you became aware of during your check-in in a Mindfulness Fertility Log:

What thoughts went through my mind before/during/ after the check-in?

_____

_____

What feelings did I connect with?

_____

_____

What sensations did I notice?

_____

_____

Bringing attention to the thoughts, feelings and sensations that came up during the exercise can help deepen your connection with your mindfulness practice. Noticing any positive changes can be particularly supportive in the beginning stages of a daily practice. Why would we change if we don't remember why we're doing it?

## Fertility-related Stress

Understanding stress within a more integrated mind–body view is not a new concept. Hippocrates, the founder of Western medicine, referred to the importance of treating the human spirit alongside the physical illness. An understanding of health problems from a mind and body perspective is commonplace in many Eastern cultures, for example, in Chinese medicine, and taking this more holistic approach is also increasing in Western medicine. Mind–body programmes are being included as part of treatment in more and more fertility clinics, as consultants perceive the benefit of having a mind–body approach to fertility care.

The idea of the mind and body as two separate entities was first expounded by René Descartes, the 17th-century French philosopher, and subsequently adopted into medicine; the body required treatment by the physician and compliance by the patient. During this period, anything associated with an enquiring mind with regards to health choices and one's overall well-being was perceived to fall into the 'guidance' role of the religious orders, unless there were severe psychiatric symptoms that required medical intervention. Though less prevalent today, there can sometimes be an over-focus on the medical and pharmaceutical treatments and protocols for fertility without due attention or support being given to the psychological and psychosomatic stress associated with fertility treatment. In the absence of receiving or seeking emotional and psychological support, it is understandable that fertility patients develop stress about being stressed – 'What's wrong with me, why can't I cope like everyone else? I can't stand this feeling.'

According to some research, our psychological well-being also impacts on pregnancy rates. One study undertaken showed that women who participated in a stress management mind–body programme prior to or during IVF treatment had a 52 per cent pregnancy success rate compared with 20 per cent for women who did not participate in the programme.[4] One hundred and forty-three women under the age of 40 took part in the research. Dr Alice Domar, one of the authors of the study, also outlined further research explaining the benefits of interventions that included a minimum of five counselling sessions, education and group support to reduce depression and anxiety and increase life satisfaction.[5] Also, a review of research that examined 14 studies relating to outcomes showed that those who received psychosocial with psychological support treatment had a 42 per cent higher chance of a pregnancy compared with those in the control group.[6]

In contrast, previous research stated that 'pre-treatment emotional distress was not associated with treatment outcome after a cycle of assisted reproductive technology'.[7]

Undertaking a comparison of literature between 1980 and 2007 on the relationship between stress and reproductive outcomes, researchers have concluded that, 'biological evidence points to an immune–endocrine disequilibrium in response to stress and describes a hierarchy of biological mediators involved in a stress trigger to reproductive failure'.[8] The research also pointed out that each individual responds to stress differently.

Further to the above, research presented at the European Society of Human Reproduction and Embryology (ESHRE) 2015 annual conference reported the findings of a study of 401 couples in the US who were monitored over 12 months, where the first physical levels of stress were measured in women trying to achieve pregnancy, to ascertain any causal effect. Levels of the stress hormones cortisol and alpha-amylase were measured in women trying to conceive. The findings concluded that 'higher levels of stress as measured by salivary alpha-amylase are associated with a longer time-to-pregnancy and an increased risk of infertility'.[9] According to the findings reported in ESHRE's journal *Human Reproduction*, the women with the highest alpha-amylase levels were on average 29 per cent less likely to get pregnant during each cycle than the women with the lowest levels.

Similarly, research undertaken in the UK observed 274 women, aged 18–40, and assessed salivary stress biomarkers over six cycles or until pregnant and concluded that, 'Stress significantly reduced the probability of conception each day during the fertile window, possibly exerting its effect through the sympathetic medullar pathway'.[10]

During times of 'fight-or-flight' responses, alpha-amylase produces what are known as catecholamines, which according to the researchers, seem to reduce blood flow, thus slowing down and negatively affecting the passage of the fertilized egg to the uterus. 'That may mean the egg does not get there in time to implant', according to the director of research, Germane Buck Louis, PhD.[11] Stress also impacts on the hormones responsible for controlling sperm production, negatively affecting both sperm quality and also reducing sperm count.[12]

Whether there is a direct correlation between stress and decreased pregnancy chances or not, it is reasonable to recommend that individuals and couples work towards supporting themselves on a physical, psychological and emotional level. This is necessary to ensure that they are experiencing their optimum physical and mental health to manage the challenging process of treatment and to ensure that their mind health and general well-being are not significantly compromised before, during or after the process.

# 1. Effects of Repeated Stress on the Body

Hypothalamus
(hidden inside brain)

Pituitary

Adrenals

**Repeated Stress Reaction & How it affects the Body**

**Hypothalamus** in Brain signals
↓
**Sympathethic Nervous System**
↓
**Fight, flight, freeze or flee**
↓
Signals **Pituitary gland** to release adrenocorticotropic hormone (ACTH) which stimulates the adrenal glands
↓
**Adrenal glands release stress hormones – Cortisol & Epinephrine (adrenaline)**
↓

| | |
|---|---|
| Increase/ decrease appetite | Increased blood pressure |
| Blood sugar imbalance | Increased heart rate |
| Slower digestive system & IBS | Suppressed Immune System |
| | Increased inflammation & muscle tension |

Female
Reproductive
System

**Psychological:**
Decreased Serotonin/ Dopamine
Worrying thoughts/ anxious mind/ irritability
Low mood or depressed & inability to concentrate
Sleep deprivation
Exhaustion or hyperarousal
Reduced Oxytocin released by Pituitary – 'bonding' hormone (may feel distant/ disassociated)

**Reproductive System Affected:**

**Female Fertility**
Changes in GnRH secretion
Decreased FSH and LH secretion
Reduced sexual drive
Reproductive hormone Imbalance – Estrogen dominance & progesterone deficiency
Decreased Thyroid function (energy production & hormone balance)
Irregular menstruation

**Male Fertility**
Loss of libido
Imbalance of testosterone
Lower sperm production
Erectile Dysfunction

## 2. Effects of Repeated Relaxation Response on the Body

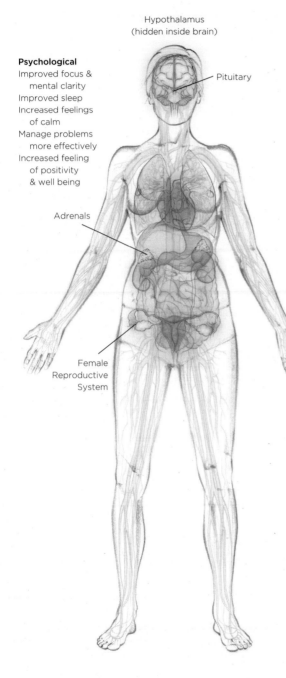

Hypothalamus
(hidden inside brain)

Pituitary

**Psychological**
Improved focus &
  mental clarity
Improved sleep
Increased feelings
  of calm
Manage problems
  more effectively
Increased feeling
  of positivity
  & well being

Adrenals

Female
Reproductive
System

**Repeated Relaxation Response
& How it affects the body**

**Hypothalamus** in Brain signals
↓
**Parasympathic System Activated**
↓
**Repeated Relaxation Response**

**Mind Health**
Increased GABA, calming
  neurotransmitter
Relaxes nervous system
Balanced dopamine
  neurohormones increases
  feelings of well-being
Balanced seretonin uplifts mood
↓

**Body Health**
Supports gland function
  regulation
Lowers heart rate & blood
  pressure
Reduces release of Cortisol thus
  blood sugar balanced
Increased antibodies in immune
  systems

**Benefits to fertility**
Supports hormone GNrH, FSH and
  LH balance in men required for
  normal sperm production
Supports hormone balance of
  oestrogen, progesterone & FSH
  and LH in women required for
  ovulation
Supports normal thyroid
  functioning
Increased release of oxytocin
  'bonding' hormone
Healthy libido & sexual functioning
Healthy mind supports a healthy
  lifestyle

Fertility problems are more than a physical concern and can have a far and wide-reaching impact on a person's life:

- They can impact on relationships: nurturing your relationship with your partner throughout treatment and beyond is particularly important as the strain of trying for a baby can lead to self-blame and a lack of desire for intimacy. Having 'fertility-free zones' in the home and dates without fertility discussions are recommended. In addition, feelings of envy and jealousy may grow towards friends and colleagues who seem to take getting pregnant for granted. This can lead to a withdrawal from social occasions and result in feelings of isolation.
- They can lead to a reduced libido. There is nothing spontaneous about timed sexual intercourse!
- They can affect financial stability: an IVF cycle can cost from 5,000 euros to 12,000 dollars depending on which clinic or country you have treatment in. Couples may need to undertake several IVF cycles before (and they may not be successful) achieving a pregnancy.
- They can challenge religious beliefs, for example, 'Why are we being chosen to be treated this way; what did we do wrong? I prayed so much and it hasn't worked this time and I no longer have faith.'
- They can damage career prospects as daily injections and hospital or doctor consultations become difficult to juggle within the daily demands of a work environment.

Taking practical, positive steps to relieve fertility-related stress can help to reduce the symptoms. By bringing your whole self to your fertility journey, you gain the strength to self-regulate difficult emotions and use your innate mind–body wisdom for a more self-empowered experience.

## Five Helpful Steps to Ease Fertility Stress

### Step 1: Understand your Triggers

- Identify your stressors: which part of the fertility assessment and treatment process in particular is making you feel most stressed?
- Contemplate the following questions: Where am I when I'm feeling stressed? What am I doing? Who am I with? Where possible, reduce these interactions during treatment. Remember, 'friends for a reason, friends for a season and friends for a lifetime' – is this the friend for this season?
- What helpful changes could you make? List people, places, hobbies and things that increase your feelings of well-being. What did you enjoy doing before dealing with fertility problems? These are often the things we let go of first when we're feeling under pressure. When/where are the times you don't feel stressed? Note and increase these occasions.
- Which parts of the infertility testing and treatment process are in your control? Which parts of the infertility testing and treatment process are outside of your control? Would it help or hinder if you let go of responsibility for those aspects of the treatment outside of your control?

### Step 2: Increase your Mindfulness Practice

* Set aside time each morning and evening for mindfulness sitting practices. Mindfulness supports stress reduction and generates space to 'check-in' with your inner self; what is the emotional tone today and how can I take care of myself? Allowing your feelings and thoughts to be present without trying to figure them out or analyse them can help to centre your mind and body at the beginning and end of your day.

### Step 3: Write a Journal

* Writing a journal during times of stress has been shown to slow down the mind, provide clarity of thought and reduce the physiological effects of trauma.[13]
* The act of writing (not typing on your laptop!) accesses your left brain, which is analytical and rational. It also frees your right brain to create intuitive solutions to problems, process difficult feelings and nurture a deeper understanding of your problems and yourself.

### Step 4: Keep a Positive Ledger

* During times of difficulty, it is easy to lose focus on the areas of our lives that are working. Generating positive feelings – joy, gratitude, contentment, etc. – tends to create an 'upward spiral', helping to increase feelings of well-being. We can keep a positive ledger by noticing three things each day that we are grateful for, proud of or enjoyed, for example, a telephone call with a friend, a compliment

affirming our work from our boss or a quiet moment with a cup of herbal tea.

## Step 5: Be Prepared for Tests and Consultant Feedback

- You can support a reduction in stress by preparing for treatment consultations in advance, writing down questions beforehand and taking notes during consultations. It can also help to take along your partner or a friend to clarify what was said during your appointment. This is particularly true if you have experienced a negative outcome as naturally it can be difficult to take in medical facts when feeling emotionally vulnerable.
- Some people find preparing a CD with their favourite mindfulness and relaxation tracks helps them during scans and medical procedures such as injections, preparing for egg retrieval or for embryo transfer.
- It may also help to arrange a pre-visit to theatre to become emotionally prepared before procedures such as egg retrieval, intrauterine insemination (IUI), testicular sperm extraction (TESE), etc. Without fear of the unknown, you can become more present and less anxious. This can sometimes be facilitated by a nurse or theatre assistant. Some clinics also include theatre visits as part of their information open days. However, if the clinic is situated in a hospital this may not be possible.

## Mindfulness-based Stress Reduction for Fertility

> And now here is my secret, a very simple secret: it is only with the heart that one can see rightly, what is essential is invisible to the eye.
>
> Antoine de Saint-Exupéry, *The Little Prince*

Mindfulness increases our ability to gain more internal space from problems and stressors, and consequently relax, even if faced with a personal crisis, such as infertility, when we would usually lose the serenity of our mind and body. When faced with the challenge of living with fertility problems, it is natural to sometimes feel negative emotions such as sadness, grief, stress, irritability and frustration. Mindfulness supports you not to be overwhelmed by these feelings.

Thinking about your hoped-for child is often accompanied by mixed feelings; longing and sadness can quickly give way to a preoccupation with strategies to bring this dream to fruition. However, the more we get caught in this 'doing' mode, the more we can become driven by demanding ways of thinking, for example, 'We *should* do this'; 'We *need* to do more'; 'We *ought* to follow this treatment approach now.' While it is important to plan, this way of thinking can progressively bring our attention further away from ourselves and, as a result, we begin to lose the ability to make balanced, wise decisions. Instead we increase the stream of worrying, anxious thoughts, which in turn lead to more feelings of low mood and stress.

Mindful awareness of moments in the here and now also helps us to let go of self-blaming thoughts relating to the distant and not-so-distant past – for example, 'Why didn't I try for children sooner?' or 'Why did I waste so much time with that relationship that didn't work?' – as well as worrying thoughts about the future: 'What if we never have children?' or 'What will I do if my partner leaves me?' Mindfulness cultivates a capacity to observe these thoughts as simply thoughts, rather than facts that we react to; for example, you begin to argue and find fault with your partner because deep down you believe he/she will leave you anyway. By acknowledging the presence of self-blaming thoughts rather than believing them, we don't generate the tension and painful feelings that are usually associated with such anxious thinking.

Being open to the energy and healing that can emerge with mindfulness practice requires a disengagement from our busy minds. Much of our daily life relies on the ability to critically analyse the choices available to us before making a decision: shall I choose this clinic or that one? Is it better to take route A or route B home from work? Do I assert myself in this situation or not? In contrast, mindfulness requires that we simply become a human 'being' rather than our usual human 'doing' self. Cultivating an attitude of being more 'present' increases with practice through such things as mindfulness meditations. We don't need to aim to 'relax more' or relax better!

Increasing mindful awareness brings more stillness to the psychological, physiological and emotional experience of facing fertility problems and replaces the all too frequent self-blaming inner critic with a more compassionate and accepting inner friend. Mindfulness offers us a well of resources to draw from on the fertility journey, with an understanding that 'You cannot draw from an empty well.'

The 'Relaxation Response'

The benefits of eliciting the 'Relaxation Response' were first expressed by Dr Herbert Benson of the Benson-Henry Institute for Mind Body Medicine at Harvard Medical School.[14] Interestingly, Dr Benson undertook his research in the very room that Walter Cannon had previously researched and outlined the physiological impact of the 'fight-or-flight response' many years before. Benson explains that when the body reacts to stress, it releases hormones – adrenaline and non-adrenaline – to increase our heart rate, breathing rate and blood pressure. This is necessary to prepare our body for a rapid response and ultimately for our survival. However, instead of relying on the 'fight-or-flight' response to run from attacking bears in prehistoric times, we are now relying on it routinely when the traffic lights turn red and other such 'emergencies'! As outlined previously, this impacts negatively on our body and our reproductive system (see page 34). Conversely, Dr Benson and his fellow researchers outlined an equally important survival mechanism: our body's ability to 'heal and rejuvenate', which he described as 'the Relaxation Response – an inducible, physiologic state of quietude'.

The benefits of inducing the Relaxation Response include:

* a more focused mind
* lowered blood pressure and heart rate, and more balanced hormone levels, whether trying to achieve pregnancy naturally or with assisted fertility treatment, balanced hormones enhance the chances of a successful pregnancy

- a deep sense of relaxation, which supports physical health
- a more proactive approach to our own health, healing and wellness.

Furthermore, medical conditions such as infertility benefit from stress reduction and it is a cost-free healing approach!

There are a variety of ways to elicit the Relaxation Response. They include:

- meditation and breathwork (for example, mindfulness)
- creative visualization
- Progressive Muscle Relaxation (tensing each muscle group in our bodies for the count of five and releasing for the count of five from our head to our feet – see page 153
- Restorative exercise, for example, hatha yoga, tai chi or qi gong.

## Writing as Therapy

'This being human is a guest-house.
Every morning a new arrival.
A joy, a depression, a meanness,
Some momentary awareness comes
As an unexpected visitor.
Welcome and entertain them all!'

Rumi, 13th-century poet

Keeping a journal is both therapeutic and pragmatic; it provides a space to express difficult emotions and, at times, to reason with the part of us that feels overwhelmed. This can lead to new ideas and possible solutions. It helps us to access our 'wise mind' by bringing balance to our emotional and rational self during all-important decision-making moments. Journaling also gives the writer permission to give full expression to conflicting internal views, working through problems and accessing the subconscious mind. For those of us who tend to overthink our problems, writing can help to quieten the mind, contributing towards clarity of thought and lessening tension in the body.

Barack Obama as US President outlined the value he placed on writing in a diary, describing it as 'an important exercise to clarify what I believe, what I see, what I care about and what my deepest values are.'[15] In creating a space to write, we can access parts of ourselves that may not be finding a voice in the automatic pilot of our day-to-day lives. Writing can help to shine a light on our deepest understandings and what we truly believe at the core of ourselves. This can often get lost in the expectations we have of ourselves or those imposed externally, for example by family, friends or society.

Susan Sontag, the influential author and film-maker, described how we can evolve personally if journaling on a regular basis: 'In the journal, I do not just express myself more openly than I could to any person; I create myself'.[16] The power of the pen was also valued by Charles Darwin, Thomas Jefferson and Winston Churchill, who all recorded their thoughts and ideas in company and privately with their notebook and pen.

Whether you are engaging with a natural-health practitioner or deciding to embark on assisted fertility treatment and making decisions regarding treatment options – IUI versus IVF; IVF versus donation; a natural approach versus assisted reproductive treatment – journaling can help you to connect with your emotions and take a more solution-focused approach when faced with many options. It is often in the moments of stillness or in journaling that we can access our intuition and, therefore, our wise mind choices.

As we have between 40,000 and 60,000 thoughts in any 24-hour period and can express up to 58 emotions at any one time, it can only be beneficial to be inspired by the influential thinkers of our age and take a pen to paper!

Writing our uninterrupted thoughts and feelings is a way of accessing our own truth rather than unquestionably following the suggestions of others, even when those suggestions are well-meaning. For patients undertaking fertility treatment, accessing deeply held thoughts, feelings or values supports the choices being made.

### A Ten-step Journaling Guide

1. In the spirit of self-care, buy yourself a really special journal to take you through your days dealing with fertility issues.
2. It is about writing rather than typing so please put away the laptop!
3. Try to write your journal at the same time each day, as this will be habit-forming.
4. Write continuously for three pages and then stop . . . to be continued.
5. Park your inner critic. This exercise is not about having the correct spelling or grammar; it is about thoughts, feelings and musings about your fertility-related plans and journey, and all that that entails. Keep writing and writing and writing; no editing required.
6. You can write about your dreams of having a baby, what it has meant to have to keep trying and how you find the process. You can include your thoughts and feelings about fertility tests coming up, what's going well, what is challenging, how your relationship is, etc. It is your space to write all your hopes, fears, challenges and resolutions.
7. Remember, you can journal to gain a deeper insight or use it as an emotional dustbin!
8. You can use the written word or visual images to express your thoughts and feelings at this time. It is all about letting go of thought control.
9. If something is too difficult to write about, you could try to write about it in the third person. It gives you another perspective, for example, if I was a good friend of mine observing this, what would I say or do?
10. Write from your intuitive self. Beneath our expectations and those we believe others have of us is our true voice. Writing without judgement allows us to access our inner voice of truth or our intuitive self. You may be surprised to find that it's not always what you expected.

## Journaling to Heal

People who engage with expressive writing report feeling happier and less negative than before writing. Similarly reports of depressive symptoms, rumination and anxiety tend to drop in the weeks or months after writing about emotional upheavals.

> Professor James Pennebaker, author and Professor of
> Psychology at the University of Texas

As it gives voice to our feelings, journaling can help us to gain a deeper self-understanding and improve communication within couple relationships. Having clarity of mind helps us to express our needs assertively rather than communicating them in an aggressive (for example, being critical or manipulative) or passive-aggressive (for example, sulking) way, which leads to healthier ways of relating and responding to each other. Differences can be explored and clarified rather than accumulating internally until feelings of resentment take over. The journal can serve as a vehicle for emotional catharsis, while also limiting the impact of unresolved issues as you begin to see clearly when you are responding to present situations from the perspective of past fears or hurts. An example could be bringing the fear of a previously unsuccessful cycle into a new and different treatment approach: 'This can't possibly work because it didn't work last time.'

Writing about a specific distressing event is best carried out within a time-limited approach, otherwise it can deepen the sense of distress rather than helping to resolve it. It can also prompt more unhelpful strategizing or ruminating on the experience rather than supporting your healing.

You may find yourself feeling vulnerable, sad or stressed during the writing process. It is essential to stop as you need to and manage your distress, perhaps by taking a mindful walk or nurturing yourself by listening to a relaxing track from your favourite CD, before returning to the journaling. It is important to ensure that you are balancing the benefits of journaling with your own self-care. It is also helpful if you have someone who you can turn to for support, for example your partner or a good friend. Some individuals prefer to do this journaling work as part of their therapeutic process with a counsellor or psychotherapist.

As stressful events are also accompanied by unpleasant feelings and thinking patterns, we often try to suppress them with avoidance or distraction. However, this can lead to more symptoms, for example, if I ask you not to think of a pink elephant what happens? One usually appears in our imagination! Likewise, in our vain attempts to decrease our upsetting thoughts, we invite more of them, which can leave us feeling mentally exhausted and more confused. Journaling can provide a release from pent-up emotions and ruminating thinking styles. Facing our distress and directly contextualizing our experience in writing allows us to let go of all the associated fear, thoughts and feelings. It also clears the path for new experiences.

Research has shown that journaling about stressful or traumatic events has been shown to benefit the individual both psychologically and physically.[17] The benefits of expressive journal writing in the long-term include:

* improved functioning in biochemical markers relating to the immune system[18] (significant for many women with fertility problems)
* improved liver function
* lowered stress levels
* an increase in positive mood and emotions
* an overall increased sense of well-being
* reduced symptoms of low mood
* reduced blood pressure
* improved physical performance
* improved memory function
* reduced visits to the GP
* assistance with pain management
* improved sleep
* reduced physiological symptoms relating to stress.[19]

Journaling can also be a helpful exercise during times of transition, for example, if ending a particular fertility treatment, such as IVF or IUI, and moving on to other considerations, such as egg or sperm donation. Exploring what this means to you personally and as a couple, and what it could mean to a potential child, can help you to move forward with wisdom and clarity, supporting self-empowered decision-making.

You will be asked to journal about different aspects of your fertility-related process throughout this book (exercises are marked with the following symbol: ✐ ). You will gain more awareness and healing by including some reflective writing. It is important to journal continuously even if your internal critic is busy finding fault with the content.

## Your Fertility Story

Some women and men I have worked with in a therapeutic setting have used this exercise to process their sense of loss if they have experienced a negative outcome following treatment, or if they have experienced a miscarriage. Journaling has helped them to connect and move through their stages of grief and to bring them some healing. If you are still feeling in the 'shock' phase of loss, however, it is wiser to begin the exercise after two or three weeks as you may feel too disorientated presently (see page 15).

This exercise is to help you process an emotionally charged issue. Some people find it helpful to share their insights within a therapeutic setting. It is not meant to replace your counselling support, although it can certainly add to it. Remember to have a plan in place should you become overly distressed. This can include seeking support from your partner, a friend or within a therapeutic environment. You can stop the exercise if you feel unable to continue. You can also decide to begin again. If you feel completely stuck and unable to move forward, you may wish to work through the issue with a fertility counsellor or medical professional first.

This exercise is not about how you write, so you don't need to correct grammar or spelling. It is about writing your deepest thoughts and the feelings that surface in relation to your fertility experience. The goal is to be fully present; as honest and true as you possibly can. It is not advisable to continue to write after the 20–30 minutes allocated for this exercise, as if you go too deeply into the process it can feel excessive. Be guided by your intuition rather than pushing yourself past a point that feels safe. Be mindful of the self-care aspect of this work.

This is also your personal work and though you may wish to share it, only do so with someone that will hold and respect the content being expressed. Otherwise, you may feel more vulnerable and exposed and your inner voice of expression will be silenced as you defend against further exploration. This is a confidential and important date with your truth.

* Find a quiet space where you are not likely to be disturbed or distracted.
* Write for 20–30 minutes each day over four days using the steps below to guide you.
* If you find the exercise too distressing, leave it and return when it feels more manageable.

**Journal Activity: Use the following steps to deepen your process of discovery** 🖊

*Day 1:*
What is your fertility-related story? Write about the facts first. Describe your fertility-related problems so far.

*Day 2:*
Now fully explore how it has affected you in your thoughts, feelings and what you do. Write freely with complete abandon without self-judgement or editing.

*Day 3:*

Write about how struggling with fertility impacts on your relationships. What arises for you? Are any of these feelings familiar? Does it remind you of similar feelings you held in the past? What do you believe about yourself or your partner because of your fertility experience?

*Day 4:*

What have you realized about yourself writing this? What positive learning can you move forward with? What can you do now to take care of yourself into the future? If you can't connect with the last question, begin with: if I was taking care of myself, I would . . . How can I relate differently to my partner, my fertility-related experience and myself?

Some people like to have an ending ritual by placing the contents of the journal in a fire and symbolically letting go of difficult feelings and thoughts. However, be careful with this; one couple reported feeling a great sense of freedom until the wind changed direction in their garden and they were left scrambling for ways to quench the ever-increasing flame!

There are several junctions during your fertility stages that would gain from some reflective consideration. You can use your journal to connect to deeper personal insights and to explore your fertility-related options and what they may mean for you.

Before beginning each day's journaling, you may wish to start with some self-reflective mindfulness practice or other self-caring exercise. The meditation below can be a supportive way to connect with your journaling discoveries.

## Mindfulness Self-enquiry Meditation

Mindfulness recognizes that we often become distracted by the thoughts that run through our minds. Self-enquiry is about connecting beyond the mind chatter and agenda-making self. It provides a space to reflect and listen closely to your inner voice in advance of your journaling. You can also access this sense of true self in nature, love or at other times, for example, when listening to a moving piece of music. It is the moment when you feel your true identity rather than the version of yourself that you present to the world (for example; sister, partner, friend, colleague or patient). This is the 'I' at the centre of you, beyond fear or worry.

Use this exercise to connect directly with your experience and observe what is happening deep within. This can help you feel more embodied before you begin the journaling process and support you in concentrating on what's really important.

- Begin by sitting or lying in a comfortable position, knowing that you will be doing this exercise for 20–30 minutes. Take time to become comfortable and settled in a posture that you are likely to find easy to maintain. As you begin, just take a moment to thank yourself for committing the time and space to your self-care in this way. Gently ease your way into the feelings and thoughts relating to your day by focusing on the gentle in-breath and out-breath. Notice how your thoughts, feelings and sensations reflect the tone of your day. Just allow them to arise from within and aim to attach no judgement or appraisal of them.

◆ As you settle into the exercise, gently focus your attention back on the breath, following its natural flow. Notice the breath as it travels towards your abdomen and how your stomach gently rises on the inhale and gently releases on the exhale.

Each time your thoughts or feelings become your focus, use the following guide to return to your breath:

Notice – my thought or feeling
Allow – my thought or feeling
Let go – of my thought or feeling
Return – to my breath

◆ Feel into your breath, relaxing your abdomen and filling your lungs. Focus on the present moment – this breath 'in' now and this breath 'out' now. Stay with the breath in this way for some minutes. Breathing begins to calm the mind and settles the nervous system. Taking time to be present to our breath is taking time to be present to our well-being.

◆ Now we gently withdraw our focus from our breath and give the sensations in our body some attention. Scan your body slowly from bottom to top, noticing and being with any feelings that arise moment to moment. These may be physiological sensations or emotional in tone. They may relate to the events of the day, your thoughts or some distant memory. Just be with the feeling as it calls your attention. You may also notice that you have thoughts evaluating these sensations. Again, just notice these thoughts and observe them as you would clouds passing in the sky.

Withdraw your focus from the story of these thoughts and back to your feelings and sensations.

- Begin to explore these feelings by focusing on any strong or difficult-to-be-with emotions. Notice how present this feeling is and where you notice it in your body or mind. Before you move forward, ask yourself: is this okay for me to continue? If your intuitive self resists moving forward, acknowledge this and return your focus to your breath rising and falling until you feel centred once again. You can continue to explore this during another exercise or when you feel emotionally safe to do so. If you feel emotionally centred enough to continue, just notice and name this feeling, this sensation and this thought, allowing them to come and go, to be present and fade.

- To end this exercise, bring your focus of attention to your whole being as you attend to your in- and out-breaths. Imagine the breath moving from the top of your head all the way down your body and out of your feet. As you breathe out, imagine the breath moving all the way up and out of your body. Gain a sense of your body as a whole, with your full top-to-bottom 'inhale' and full bottom-to-top 'exhale' breaths. After several breaths like this, gently take your attention back to your present moment and when you're ready begin your journaling exercise. Choose how you manage the journaling, for example, are you particularly vulnerable today? How much can you challenge yourself today with your journaling exercise? What do you need to do for yourself once you have completed it?

- You may notice that in your still moments, your mind continues to call your attention. You may drift into the business of the mind as it strategizes, comments or judges, plans or observes. You may find yourself being drawn into dreaming about the future or the past. You may notice your thoughts are charged with the events of your day. Our thoughts can have a very strong pull. Just notice these thoughts rather than connecting with the vast content. See your thoughts as lanes of traffic: coming and going; stronger and busier; less demanding and spaced somewhat. Just observe the thoughts rather than connecting with the content.

- Strong feelings such as fear or stress may carry many thoughts with them. Face them rather than resist them, allow them to come and go without analysis or judgement (for example, why am I thinking this way? What is this feeling about?). By allowing them to be present without reacting, we often experience an acceptance of where we are just now, in this moment, leading to fewer extreme feelings of resistance. As we notice the thoughts, feelings and sensations come and go, grow stronger and disappear, we become more accepting. With less resistance comes more equanimity.

## The Physiological Impact of Fertility Treatment

When you begin your journey to enhanced fertility, you may visit natural-health practitioners and, if you are over 30, you may also quite quickly engage with assisted fertility treatment. This involves coming to terms with all the fertility-related medical language and tests you may need to undertake, which can be daunting. Chapter 3 outlines the different medical procedures involved in assisted fertility treatment and will gently guide you through the process.

Whether you are going through natural fertility support or are undertaking IUI, IVF or donor treatment, it is not uncommon to feel stressed and fearful. Research has shown that almost 40 per cent of women prior to assisted fertility treatment express symptoms of clinical depression and/or anxiety, compared to 4 per cent in the average population.[20]

While mindfulness cannot help you in determining your outcome, it can help to relieve the physiological impact of going through investigative tests and other procedures, such as testing with ovulation kits, taking pregnancy tests, TESE, scans, injections, egg retrieval, embryo transfers, etc. Practising the 'body scan' exercise below can help you to remain present in your body rather than being carried away by fearful thoughts or challenging feelings before, or during, tests and medical procedures. This can support a reduction in physical tension and also aid the healing process on both an emotional and physical level.

## The Body Scan

The body scan is a grounding and reconnecting exercise that can help to restore a sense of wholeness. It is ideal in advance of medical procedures or in the days leading up to a pregnancy test. The body scan allows you to come home to your body, bringing balance to both body and mind.

The body scan can help you to manage sensations as they arise rather than being overwhelmed by them (being 'rigid with fear'), and also become more accepting of 'what is' rather than resisting the physical experience with your thoughts and feelings, and thus magnifying them. As a result, an ultrasound becomes simply a scan, rather than all the thoughts and corresponding feelings that are associated with the scan.

Some people report feeling embarrassed or disempowered during more intrusive internal examinations at reproductive clinics. This can be particularly true for adult survivors of sexual abuse. With the body scan, you can experience a reconnection to self rather than disassociating or shutting down. By letting things be, knowing that any discomfort or pain is helping to achieve the goal of having a baby and will soon pass, any additional tension is released. Though it does not feel natural to respond to pain or discomfort in this way, doing so supports the recovery and healing process. The body scan may also help to increase calmness and psychological well-being during the two-week wait before undertaking another pregnancy test.

Aim to scan your body daily and practise inhabiting your body rather than living in your thoughts. Increasing your body awareness will lead to fewer feelings of disassociation or 'out-of-body experiences' during your natural or assisted fertility treatment.

* Sit comfortably supported in a chair or lying down on a yoga mat or on your bed (remembering that the purpose is not to fall asleep!). Ensure that you are warm and comfortable. Choose a quiet area where you are unlikely to be disturbed and allow your eyes to close gently.

* Take some deep breaths in and out. Begin to connect with the sensation of the breath entering and leaving your body. Now, take several deep breaths and feel your body as a whole form – from the top of your head to the soles of your feet. Become aware of what it feels like to connect to the chair or bed beneath you.

* Now bring your awareness to the physical sensations in your body, allowing any sensations to be present. Notice the sensation of touch: how do your clothes feel against your skin, your shoes connecting to the ground if sitting? Breathe normally as you connect with the sensations of touch or pressure. On each breath, take yourself a little deeper into your body.

* Remind yourself that you just need to be present to this moment, right now. Let go of any thoughts or desires to be different – to be less stressed or healthier, for example. Instead, as best you can, begin to focus your attention on any sensations present in your left foot and where it connects with your footwear or with the floor. Connect deeply to these sensations or lack of sensations. Feel into the toes separately, and then into the sole of the foot, moving slowing on to the Achilles tendon before focusing on the left ankle and then on the top of the foot. Notice any heat, cold or numb feelings. Notice pins and needles, comfort or discomfort. If you can't feel any sensations, just be present to that.

* Now bring your awareness into your lower left leg and any sensations detected, as you remain present to the sensations that arise. Notice how the calf and shin connect with your knee. Now focus on the knee area and gently move

your focus to the lower thigh and then sense how the top of the leg connects with the hips. Let your awareness focus on this connection.

- If your mind has wandered with thoughts, gently bring your focus back to your in- and out-breaths and then take your attention back to moving down the left leg and into the sole of your left foot, before moving your attention across to the sensations in the right foot, soles, toes, ankle and where it connects to its support with the Achilles tendon and right ankle. Let your awareness focus on the sensations on the lower calf and knee before resting on the right thigh and its connection into the right hip.

- Now have some gentle awareness of the sensations in the pelvic and reproductive area. Become mindful of any sensations or feelings associated with this area. Should your mind wander into thoughts, just notice the tone of these thoughts and gently refocus your attention away from them and on to the in- and out-breaths. Bring some expansive breaths and kind attention to your pelvic and reproductive area as you gently breathe in 'calm' and let go of any unwelcome tension in this area on the out-breath. Imagine that each breath is bringing a deeper healing to your reproductive area; gently and kindly bring a compassionate awareness to this area. Take a few minutes to feel the sensations fully as you breathe in and out.

- Leaving the awareness of the pelvic area, bring your attention to sensations present in the lower abdomen, becoming aware without judgement of the changing patterns of sensations in the abdomen and digestive area as you gently breathe in, and out.

● Now begin to bring the focus of your awareness to the chest area as it rises and falls with each breath. Notice any expansive or restrictive sensations as your diaphragm rises and falls like waves on the sea, gently moving upwards and fading away, upwards and fading away.

● Gently refocus your attention on the lower-back area and how it connects with your supportive breath. Move your attention of focus up the spine area and out towards the rib cage and lung area, before moving to the upper areas of the back and shoulder blades. Notice any comfort or discomfort in these areas, feeling the sensations as you gently move up and out from the spine. Become aware of your breath rising and falling, entering and leaving your body as you focus attentively on each sensation.

● When you are ready, take the focus of your attention away from your upper back and shoulder blades on to the fingertips moving down into the palms of your left hand. Then connect to any sensations in your lower and upper arm and rest your attention on any sensations in your shoulders.

● Now take your attention to the fingertips on your right hand, palm, lower right arm and upper arm as it connects to your shoulder blade. Are there any sensations or feelings present when you focus on this area? Gently note any sensations before moving your attention to the top of your head, your forehead, temples and down into your jaw and mouth area. Connect deeply with any sensations in your entire head area. Notice any sensations resonating in these areas, letting go of any thoughts that may arise and taking the focus back to the breath . . . in and out, rising and falling.

* Now bring awareness to the physical sensations of the body as a whole with all its feelings, thoughts and emotions. Be present to your whole body, taking a deep breath in and scanning from the top of your head to your feet, and being aware of your body as a whole on the exhale.
* Take three full 'whole-body' awareness breaths in and out.

When you notice that your mind has wandered, gently bring your focus back to the sensations in your body with the breath acting as your anchor to reconnect. It is normal for the mind to wander into thoughts, but we can gently become present to the sensations and our breath again.

You can either spend a long time on each area to really connect with your body and explore where your body holds and releases your feelings and sensations for 45 minutes daily, or you can focus on larger parts of the body for 30 minutes.

### Safe-place Visualization

It may be helpful to combine the body scan with a creative visualization exercise to support you if you experience physical discomfort during treatment or have a needle phobia. Applying mindfulness breathwork with this safe-place exercise deepens the relaxation experience.

* Begin by imagining that you are in your 'safe place' – a favourite place where you feel completely relaxed. This safe

place can be a real or imaginary place (select a suitable image to draw inspiration from).

- Close your eyes gently and visualize yourself going on a journey through your senses into your safe place. What sounds would you expect to hear in your safe place (for example, a trickling brook or leaves rustling in a wood)? Imagine these sounds surrounding you now. Take yourself more deeply into your safe place with each deep in-breath and releasing out-breath.

- As you visualize being in the centre of your safe place, imagine what smells would be present to you there. Would it be the salty air of the sea or the aroma of fresh pines from the forest? Imagine the familiar smells of your safe place being available to you now.

- As your sense of yourself in your safe place deepens, begin to notice what sensations you would feel while there. Would it be warm or cool? Are your clothes soft to the touch or are you wrapped in warmth? Explore how you feel in your safe place. Do you feel held and secure?

- Now connect to the emotional feeling in your safe place. How do you feel deep within (for example, calm or relaxed) and where in your body do you hold that feeling (for example, in the chest area)?

- Bring yourself to your safe place by connecting with each of your senses and keep breathing mindfully throughout – gentle and deep breaths in through your nose and out through your mouth, sensing each breath as you take yourself there.

- Give your safe place a name, for example 'the waterfall' or 'my bedroom', and when feeling stressed, just remind yourself to take yourself there. Your safe-place exercise can be done lying down or sitting up with your eyes open or closed.

These mindfulness and visualization practices are important to deepen our mind–body awareness of pleasant, unpleasant or neutral thoughts and feelings. By bringing your whole self to your fertility enhancement or treatment process, you won't be as easily swayed by strong feelings, sensations or thoughts as you learn to remain centred with the help of gentle mindfulness exercises. Mindfulness will also help to increase feelings of compassion towards yourself and your partner. In addition to gaining the strength to self-regulate difficult emotions, you will increasingly use your innate mind–body wisdom to experience a more self-empowered fertility journey.

There are many fertility treatment options to consider, as outlined in the following chapter, and applying mindfulness-based stress reduction skills will facilitate you to engage with your medical treatment with self-care and a sense of wholeness.

# CHAPTER 3

## *Assisted Reproductive Treatment*

......................................................................................

The wish for healing has always been half of health.

LUCIUS ANNAEUS SENECA, ROMAN
PHILOSOPHER AND STATESMAN, 65AD

......................................................................................

In general, couples have an 80 per cent chance of conceiving within 12 months if they are having regular (every two or three days) intercourse and they are under the age of 40.[1] It can be difficult to decide whether you require assisted medical fertility treatment or whether you should take into account lifestyle factors and continue trying naturally. Arming yourself with the right information generally supports wiser treatment choices and helps to make those decisions easier as you work out the physical, psychological, financial and emotional gains and losses for each option.

Medical fertility treatment will include some of the following:

* Assessing ovulation and the number and quality of oocytes available in the ovaries.
* Undertaking a sperm analysis test to assess sperm quality and function.

- Examination of the fallopian tubes and uterus with a hysterosalpingogram (HSG): an X-ray test that uses a contrast material dye to assess flow through the uterus and fallopian tubes to ascertain if there is any blockage of movement which may prevent the sperm reaching the egg to fertilize. It can also highlight any issues (polyps, for example), which may be preventing implantation to the wall of the uterus.
- A surgical examination of your pelvic region with a laparoscopy.
- Fertility drugs may be used to induce ovulation or improve hormone production.
- Surgery may be required to remove any fibroids or polyps from the uterus or endometriosis from around the fallopian tubes.
- Hormone therapy may be used to improve sperm production.
- Sometimes men will require testicular sperm extraction (TESE) to retrieve adequate numbers of sperm, to be used in in-vitro fertilization (IVF) or intracytoplasmic sperm injection (ICSI).
- Genetic diagnosis is sometimes recommended where both individuals are carriers of genetic disorders to support them having children without them developing the disease.

It is recommended that if you are under the age of 35 and have not conceived within 12 months of having regular intercourse, or you are over the age of 35 and have not conceived within six months, that you seek medical support. This may mean attending your GP in the first instance or you may wish to contact a fertility clinic and undertake some initial assessment tests, as outlined above. Remember, these are not all routine tests and it is important that you check with your clinic which of them they offer in their standard male and female fertility tests. As women are half as fertile at 40 as they were at 35, it is important to undergo the appropriate tests to determine the best course of fertility treatment to optimize your chances of success.

## Choosing a Clinic

Most fertility clinics in Europe and the United States work within a legislative framework for fertility treatment. Governing bodies such as the UK's Human Fertilisation & Embryology Authority (HFEA), the European Society of Human Reproduction and Embryology (ESHRE) and the American Society for Reproductive Medicine (ASRM) ensure that quality standards are maintained. It is helpful to gather as much information as possible about treatment options, experiences and success rates of clinics before attending for assessment.

When choosing a clinic you may wish to consider the following:

- What are the statistics for live birth rates at the clinic? This is more relevant than positive pregnancy results achieved. These can usually be found on the clinic's website.
- Are the statistics verified and are they above or below the national average (the HFEA verifies all statistics provided for UK clinics)?

- What are the costs for treatment? Is it all-inclusive? For example, is it an overall cost for an egg donation treatment, or are there likely to be additional treatment costs?
- Will treatment at this clinic be convenient? If it involves travel for each appointment, how will that work socially or in regards to work obligations? As it is a medical problem, all treatment will require some compromise in regards to day-to-day commitments, however this needs to be factored in when planning your treatment.
- Does the clinic work with a satellite clinic close to where I live? A satellite clinic may offer monitoring scans and blood tests to save you travel time. Main procedures such as assessment, egg collection, embryo transfers etc, are undertaken at the main clinic.
- Are there any online reviews of the clinic/consultant being attended?
- Will the clinic provide psychological support?
- Do you need to attend an additional healthcare professional? If taking an integrative approach to your fertility healthcare, you may attend a specialist fertility counsellor and/or nutritionist and/or complementary healthcare practitioner, for example, an acupuncturist. It is important to also consider your psychological, emotional and mind–body health needs.
- Do you need to factor time off work to attend the clinic? Sometimes (if not time limited) your fertility treatment can be scheduled to work within annual leave, for example if working as a teacher you may begin treatment during your annual leave entitlement. Of course, this is not always possible.

- Has your doctor recommended this clinic? Do they have information with regards to patient feedback on the clinic?
- Has the clinic consultant trained specifically as a fertility specialist? How long have they worked as a specialist fertility consultant?
- What are your needs with regards to a clinic?
- If you need donor treatment:
    - Is there a waiting list and if so, how long is it?
    - Does the clinic offer identifiable donation? Research shows this is helpful to consider in regards to the psychological welfare of the adult donor child and family dynamics in the long term.
- If you know anybody who has attended this clinic, what was their experience?
- If changing clinic, ask yourself: in what way do I hope the new clinic will be different? What do I need to be different? Have I communicated these needs to the clinic consultant?

Bear in mind that communicating effectively with your consultant can lead to a more self-empowered treatment process (see Chapter 8 for more guidance on this). Consultants are adept at answering patient queries. Having clarity with regards to your treatment options and considerations will help you to feel more prepared and you will experience less uncertainty in the treatment decision-making process.

Remember to leave sufficient time to process the information received at the initial appointment stage. It is also important to check-in with yourself and what your overall feeling is following your initial appointment.

**Journal Activity: Your Clinic Visit** 🖊

Journaling can help you to connect to how you feel at a deeper subconscious level. Ask yourself the following questions and then write your responses without self-editing so that you are responding from your intuitive self:

* How did I feel after attending the clinic?
* If I received challenging feedback regarding tests undertaken, how was this communicated to me?
* Did I feel heard?
* Did I feel met with regards to my medical needs?
* Did I feel met with regards to my emotional and psychological needs?
* Do I think this clinic offers sufficient expertise to treat my particular fertility problem and provide me with the treatment required?
* After this meeting, would I recommend this clinic to a friend? If so, why? If not, why not?
* Was the clinic transparent in regards to treatment costs involved?

Exploring our emotional felt sense and balancing this with the gains and losses of following a particular treatment path, or attending this clinic versus another, usually contributes towards wiser and clearer decision-making.

## The Initial Consultation

Have you written down important questions and concerns for your first consultation appointment? It is often emotionally challenging to attend a clinic for the first time and it can help in your preparation to write down some questions for the consultant. They may include:

- In regards to any recommended treatment, why this treatment option and how successful has it been for similar presenting fertility issues?
- What is the consultant's interpretation of the AMH and semen analysis results and what are the treatment options based on the results?
- How likely is a positive pregnancy with this treatment option given my AMH result and my age?
- What medication will be recommended with my treatment option and what are the likely side effects?
- What is the timeline and recommended treatment plan?

A fertility clinic will carry out a full evaluation of the individual/couple at their initial consultation. This will include a full medical history to highlight any potential problems causing the infertility and also the most effective recommended treatment plan.

The fertility consultant will undertake a detailed questionnaire and physical examination, and it is recommended that any medical records pertaining to previous fertility tests or treatment be available at this consultation (ideally forwarded in advance).

Following this, the consultant will recommend specific tests that are usually undertaken on the same day. Assessment and tests will be used to identify important points, such as detecting ovulation, assessing the fallopian tubes and the uterus to detect any problems, including blocks in the fallopian tubes, polyps or fibroids. Blood tests will be undertaken to identify any thyroid problems or anaemia and an anti-müllerian hormone (AMH) test will be carried out to ascertain egg reserve. An evaluation of the health and production of sperm will also be undertaken with a full sperm analysis. Semen analysis includes assessment of the number, quality (shape) and motility (movement) of sperm. The results are usually available within a few days of the tests and will form the basis for diagnosis and treatment.

Your initial consultation will include a questionnaire to outline the following:

- Perceived duration of infertility problem.
- Any previous tests and treatment undertaken.
- Female: menstrual and gynaecological history.
- Male: urological history and any previous sperm analysis results.
- Current medication. Any known allergies to medication.
- Previous pregnancies. Also, if this is secondary infertility: what, if any, significant health or lifestyle changes since birth of previous child.
- Frequency of sexual intercourse.
- Any sexual problems.

- Lifestyle factors including alcohol intake, smoking, recreational drugs, BMI (recommended to be between 19 and 30), exercise and general health.
- The questionnaire may also include an exploration of your beliefs relating to any specific tests or treatment, for example IVF, donor treatment, genetic diagnosis, and also your aspirations and limitations (financial or otherwise) concerning treatment.

Depending on the proposed treatment, an appointment with the fertility counsellor and/or nurse may be scheduled. The specialist fertility counsellor will explore any concerns you have and also the implications for treatment on a psychological and emotional level. If you are considering donor treatment, implications counselling will usually include information relating to the legal, social and ethical aspects of donor treatment. This is expanded upon in the donor treatment section below (see page 88). Counselling can also help to give you coping strategies to ensure that you are in optimum psychological health to manage the physical treatment being undertaken.

The fertility nurse will undertake the blood tests in addition to measuring your BMI (weight and height). She/he will also support you in understanding how to implement your treatment plan and also how to administer the injections if undertaking IVF.

## Causes of Fertility Problems

The most common causes of fertility problems include:

- Problems or failure to ovulate.
- Blocked fallopian tubes causing obstruction.
- Issues with sperm quality or inadequate numbers to reach the egg.
- Reduced egg quantity or quality (with advanced age or as a result of premature menopause).
- A result of infections in the reproductive tract.
- Endometriosis or adhesions in or around the ovaries, fallopian tubes or uterus.

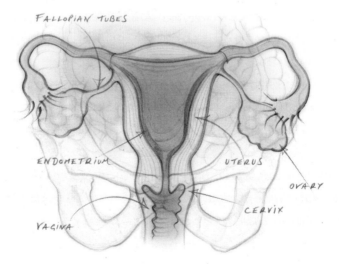

Female Reproductive System

* Uterus lining is unreceptive.
* Serious previous medical problems or treatment, for example, cancer and chemotherapy, or having had mumps as a child.
* Genetic factors.

The majority of these underlying problems can be improved with medical treatment, which happens in advance of intrauterine insemination (IUI) or IVF. Dietary changes and supplements can also help to improve symptoms.

Assisted fertility treatment will include working with a medical team consisting of a fertility consultant physician, specialist fertility nurses, sonographers, urologists, embryologists and specialist fertility counsellors. Many patients will combine this with improving lifestyle factors and engaging with psychotherapeutic and natural-health approaches, such as mindfulness stress reduction, CBT, acupuncture, etc., aimed at reducing the psychological and physiological impact of treatment and enhancing their overall health.

Although there are many potential reasons for a lack of conception, medical studies report that only 25 per cent can be categorized as 'unexplained infertility', when there is no medical explanation available to define the infertility problem.[2] However, many women achieve a successful pregnancy even with a diagnosis of unexplained infertility and so having this explanation for your problem does not mean that treatment won't succeed, although it is more difficult to treat.

## Medical Treatment Options in Assisted Fertility Treatment

Following initial tests, the best course of treatment will be decided with your consultant. It is important to remember that not all treatment is suited to every patient. Taking the time to consider if it is right for you, right for your partner and right for a potential child will support you to embrace your choices in a more empowered way. You may wish to seek the support of a specialist fertility counsellor or psychotherapist during this decision-making process.

When making decisions relating to your treatment options, the following statistics may be helpful to keep in mind:

* Intrauterine insemination is effective in over 50 per cent of women under the age of 40 within six cycles. This increases to 75 per cent with a further six cycles.[3]
* In-vitro fertilization success rates per cycle according to the latest national research are: 32 per cent for women under 35 years of age; 27.7 per cent for women aged 35–37; 20.8 per cent for women aged 38–39; and 13.6 per cent for women aged 40–42.[4]
* Couples in their twenties trying naturally have a per month success rate of 15–20 per cent. When planning for fertility treatment, keep in mind that it can be successful with the first IUI or IVF cycle, though it is more likely to take several attempts.
* Success rates with frozen sperm are similar to fresh sperm due to advanced freezing methods being used, although fertility clinics prefer to use fresh sperm in IVF cycles to

ensure there is no reduction in quantity due to the thawing process.

- Although 1 in 6 is the general statistic for infertility problems, age-related infertility affects 13–22 per cent of women at the age of 35 and 24–45 per cent of women aged 40.[5]
- Contrary to the common myth that it impacts on women more than men, infertility problems are attributed equally: 40 per cent female-related problems, 40 per cent male-related problems and 20 per cent attributed to combined male and female factors.

## Timed Sexual Intercourse (TSI)

If you have fertility problems due to irregular menstrual cycles, failure to ovulate or mistimed intercourse, your cycle will be monitored. Ovulation time and the optimum time for TSI will then be advised once you have undertaken regular pelvic ultrasound scans to evaluate the growing follicle and the thickness of your endometrium (womb lining). This is combined with blood tests to evaluate your hormone levels. Timed sexual intercourse is recommended every couple of days at the recommended time to optimize conception chances. This is often combined with 'ovulation induction' which uses fertility drugs, such as clomifene, letrozole or tamoxifen, to stimulate the development of follicles in the ovaries. You are then given a human chorionic gonadotropin (hCG) hormonal injection to induce ovulation, with TSI planned for between 12 and 24 hours after the injection to optimize the likelihood of conception.

Some women report the side effects of taking the fertility drugs as including fatigue, nausea and headaches.

Who is it Recommended For?

Timed sexual intercourse with ovulation induction is only recommended when the man's semen analysis is normal and the woman has clear fallopian tubes and no significant ovarian problems.

## Intrauterine Insemination

Intrauterine insemination optimizes your chances of conception as it includes the insemination of specially prepared washed sperm (either thawed or fresh) in sufficient number into the uterus (womb), placed closer to the egg, at the expected ovulation time. Your ovulation time is predicted by monitoring your cycle to detect a surge in luteinizing hormone (LH), which is produced in your pituitary gland and stimulates your ovaries to release the egg. Most clinics combine this with ultrasound scans to detect follicle growth. Insemination will take place when two or three follicles are present.

If your IUI accompanies stimulated treatment, you will receive fertility drugs, such as clomiphene, or follicle-stimulating hormone (FSH) injections. This stimulates the ovaries to develop the eggs and to produce oestrogen, which prepares the uterus by thickening its lining. Once the follicles are at the appropriate size, the nurse will administer an injection of hCG, ovulation medication used for maturing eggs at the end stages. The insemination will take place within 24–48 hours of this injection.

It is important that men abstain from intercourse (ejaculation) for three days (and not longer) before producing the sperm sample to be used in IUI in order to give the optimum sample.

After treatment, normal day-to-day living and intimacy can resume, once the woman has allowed an initial restful period. Although it is possible to get pregnant after the first IUI, the chances of a positive pregnancy increase with successive treatments.

## Who is it Recommended For?

Intrauterine insemination is usually recommended if there is a low sperm count or decreased sperm mobility, or in cases where the cervical mucus is not receptive to sperm, for example, women may have received treatment for negative smear tests that resulted in reducing the number of cervical secretion glands in the cervix. It is also recommended for unexplained infertility and women who have polycystic ovary syndrome (PCOS) or mild endometriosis. Intrauterine insemination is undertaken when there are fewer than two or three follicles present and, depending on other factors, IVF may be recommended.

Intrauterine insemination is also the recommended treatment with sperm donation for single women and women in same-sex relationships. Couples and individual women will still undertake all relevant fertility tests to ascertain their levels of fertility, as they may need to consider IVF instead of IUI, depending on the test results. It is also worth noting that having a stimulated monitored cycle over a natural monitored cycle more than doubles the chances of success.

### In-vitro Fertilization

The first stage of IVF involves taking medication for two weeks, via injection or nasal spray, to suppress your natural menstruation cycle. This is followed by 10–12 days of taking ovarian-stimulating drugs in the form of FSH injections.

After taking the ovarian-stimulating drugs and being monitored throughout your cycle (via ultrasound scans), IVF involves retrieving eggs (known as egg harvesting) and fertilizing the eggs with the prepared sperm in laboratory conditions. Egg harvesting involves a process where the eggs are retrieved by inserting a needle into the ovarian follicle (clinics do this under general or local anaesthetic). The sperm and eggs are then placed in a special medium culture in a laboratory dish for fertilization. Some women will experience menstruation-like cramps and some spotting after this process.

Those eggs that have been fertilized (now called embryos) are then cultured for up to five days until they reach blastocyst stage (where the cells begin to divide). The best embryo is transferred back into the woman's uterus. This is usually Day 5 of the fertilization process.

The 'best' embryo is assessed by embryologists using microscopes and, more frequently, time-lapsed embryo imaging to select the embryos that are viable and the most likely to implant.

Embryo Transfer

For younger women undertaking their first two IVF cycles, it is common to transfer one embryo during embryo transfer – fertility consultants would generally prefer to minimize the potential of multiple births due to their associated health risks. This may be increased to two embryos if undertaking a third cycle or more of IVF.

Your cervix is prepared by washing it with sterile fluid. This is a painless procedure accompanied by a pressurized sensation. A catheter (a very thin, soft tube) is then inserted into the cervix. The most viable embryo(s) are removed from the incubator in the laboratory and passed to the doctor (via a hatch mini door to save time and distance, thus minimizing exposure). The embryo(s) are transferred via the catheter and positioned close to the top of the uterine cavity. This procedure is guided using an ultrasound scan and so can be observed on a monitor screen. You will not need to be sedated for this procedure. Contrary to some beliefs, the embryos cannot fall out, even if you sneeze or cough! A positive pregnancy happens if the embryo attaches successfully to the wall of the uterine cavity.

Following embryo transfer, it is advisable to treat yourself as though in the first trimester of pregnancy: avoid heavy or strenuous exercise and lifting heavy objects, and avoid alcohol, coffee and particular foods, such as mussels, cream cheese, etc. However, it is not necessary or generally advised to spend a day in bed after embryo transfer. Take things easy but continue to remain upright while doing so!

As with any fertility treatment, IVF may be successful on

the first attempt or it may require several treatments. It is helpful when planning your IVF treatment to have in mind how much treatment you feel is appropriate to your circumstances – physically, emotionally, financially, and with regards to your relationship. According to Resolve, the national infertility association in the US, studies show that 'women are most likely to conceive if they undergo more than two IVF cycles'.[6]

## Medication

At the initial stage, in order to ascertain the levels of fertility medications to stimulate ovulation, the clinic will undertake three important tests to determine your egg reserve. One of these tests is to ascertain the FSH level. This goes up as women advance in age and the egg follicles become less efficient.

The second test is an AMH test – a blood test used to indicate the remaining ovarian reserve (egg supply). When the result is higher, it will tend to respond better to the stimulation drugs used in IVF and result in retrieving a higher number of eggs, thus increasing the chance of a successful conception as there is more potential for embryos to be replaced. It is important to note that the AMH result does not indicate egg quality but rather potential egg quantity which, of course, increases the likelihood of embryo transfer.

According to research undertaken by Dr Richard Sherbahn, although the AMH result works on a continuum and therefore does not categorize easily, the following can be used as a guideline:[7]

| Women < 35 | AMH Blood Level |
| --- | --- |
| High (usually indicates PCOS) | Over 4.0 ng/ml |
| Normal | 1-5–4.0 ng/ml |
| Low normal range | 1.0–1.5 ng/ml |
| Low | 0.5–1.0 ng/ml |
| Very low | Less than 0.5 ng/ml |

*reproduced with permission from Dr Sherbahn (2015)

As there is usually a combination of factors to consider in fertility treatment, your consultant will assess your AMH level in the context of your overall fertility medical needs. Remember, AMH levels change with age and what may be considered low for a woman under 35 may be a positive level for a woman in her early forties. Bear in mind that the AMH result is a guideline, not the whole picture. However, it does indicate likely success with particular treatment approaches.

Most clinics interpret the AMH result along with the third test – the antral follicle count (AFC), which is the number of follicles detected using an ultrasound examination. Each 'resting' antral follicle indicates the potential for the existence of an egg to develop and release (or be retrieved in IVF). An experienced clinician can usually predict the likely potential of these developing with the appropriate ovarian-stimulation drugs and will prescribe accordingly. The AMH and FSH blood tests and AFC are usually carried out at your initial physical assessment (see page 71).

Following these tests and assessment by your clinician, ovulatory-stimulation drugs, such as gonadotropins, are administered to bring about hormone balance and increase the chances of conception. The dose of these stimulation injections will be guided by your consultant after taking into account your AMH level, FSH level and AFC, as well as your age. It is likely that the older you are and the lower your egg reserve, the higher dose of drugs may be required for you to respond to treatment. Other medications include gonadotropin-releasing hormone anologues (GnRH-a) – hormones used in a short protocol to stimulate FSH and LH production or in a longer protocol to decrease FSH and LH production. These stimulating drugs are stopped once your doctor assesses that your hormones are at the correct levels and the follicles are sufficient in size. The consultant will also assess the thickness of your womb lining. You will usually be scanned daily in your clinic or satellite clinic to determine when you need to cease taking the stimulation drugs and prepare for egg collection.

Your fertility specialist nurse will then administer the hCG 'trigger' injection to prepare the eggs for collection 36 hours later. Egg collection is a 15–20 minute procedure undertaken by the fertility gynaecologist. The embryologist assesses how many eggs have been collected and this is relayed to you when you have recovered from the anaesthetic. The prepared fresh sperm sample and the eggs are then put in a petri dish and placed in an incubator.

Medications for IVF are usually self-administered via a pen injection applicator. Some are injected just under the skin and others directly into the muscle area of the stomach. Your fertility nurse will explain exactly how to take the medication. Some of the medications, for example, GnRh-a, will be required to be taken via nasal spray. Your clinic will provide you with a comprehensive treatment plan outlining what medication to take, and when and how to take it.

## Self-care

If you are particularly nervous about taking injections, you may benefit from purchasing anaesthetic cream as it helps to numb the injection point. It is also helpful to combine your injections with some mindful breathwork techniques and become aware of 'catastrophizing' thoughts (thoughts not facts!), noticing them rather than becoming anxious due to fearful internal stories. It can also be helpful to play a relaxation CD in the background.

It is important to take gentle care of yourself and each other after egg collection and in advance of embryo transfer, usually five days later. During this five-day period, you will be taking progesterone supplements and, like other medications taken during the IVF cycle, they can be accompanied by varying degrees of side effects. Some people report experiencing headaches, mood swings or feeling physically tender, which is not surprising given the levels and function of the hormones injected. Equally, some women express that they do not experience any notable significant change. You may wish to take some days off from your regular routine around egg collection/embryo transfer time, at least for the first time that you undertake IVF treatment.

## In-vitro Fertilization with Intracytoplasmic Sperm Injection

When there is a low sperm count or poor morphology, ICSI will usually be recommended with IVF. Also, if the man needs to undergo TESE to remove the sperm from the testicles, ICSI will be recommended in order to select the best single sperm to inject into the middle of the egg by the embryologist. It may also be recommended if you have had unsuccessful IVF previously where eggs were retrieved but not fertilized or there is a high sperm DNA fragmentation level.

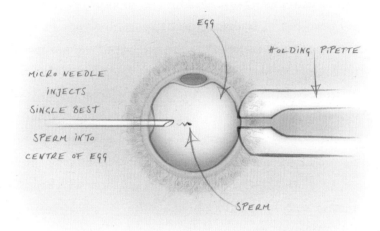

Image of ICSI – In-vitro Fertilization with
Intracytoplasmic Sperm Injection

**Journal Activity:**
**Is IVF or IUI the Right Option for Me/Us?**

Before moving forward with your treatment options, it can be helpful to consider what it will mean to you in the short, medium and long term. By exploring this more deeply, it supports you to make the best decision with the information you currently have. This leads to more clarity and less rumination, for example, 'What should I do . . . ?' 'What could I do . . . ?', 'I wish I had . . .' Explore the following questions together:

- Do you understand what is involved medically in this procedure or do you need further clarification regarding medications, how much treatment time is involved and what the likely costs may be?
- What does it mean to you to try this as a treatment option (explore practical and financial considerations and the likely emotional and psychological experience)?
- Do you have any concerns about the physical impact of treatment and also about the possible storing of embryos after treatment? Have you discussed these with your consultant?
- Have you also considered a 'Plan B'? It is helpful to have a Plan B from the outset even though you may never need to consider it if the treatment is successful. It will mean it has been thought through at a less vulnerable time, should you need it.
- What self-care/couple-care plan do you need in place?

## Egg Freezing

Egg freezing is becoming increasingly popular as an option for single women to preserve their current fertility. Women in their late twenties or in their thirties may be reflecting on their fertility and a desire to have a child but not be in a relationship, and egg freezing offers them the opportunity to preserve eggs for future insemination. As we advance in age, egg quality and quantity reduce and some women aim to prevent this by freezing their eggs. As a relatively recent treatment, you may wish to research how much experience your clinic has of egg freezing and whether they have achieved any live births.

Many clinics will recommend more than one egg retrieval cycle as egg thawing loses some eggs and, following insemination, some embryos can stop growing meaning that you are likely to have fewer embryos to transfer. Increasing the number of eggs retrieved by doing more than one cycle increases the likelihood of more embryos to transfer.

---

### Journal Activity: Considering Egg Freezing

- Why are you choosing egg freezing?
- What are the treatment options available to you?
- Does your clinic use the most modern freezing techniques (vitrification)?

---

## Egg Donation

It is a natural expectation when in a significant relationship and thinking of your future together that you see a life that will include a child or children, and that these children would most likely reflect some of your own and your partner's characteristics and genes. Therefore, moving forward with the help of donation to conceive and reach a place where you have your ideal family, albeit created in a different way, usually involves a significant process of reflection and transition.

For those who have experienced unsuccessful IVF cycles or who are overcoming miscarriage, this time of exploration can also be a time to come to terms with their sense of loss. You may need to heal from feelings of grief, such as disbelief, bargaining ('What if we'd tried this . . . ?', 'What if I'd met this consultant first . . . ?'; going over details of the past in order to try and change the present), low mood and even depression for a time, as you mourn the loss of a genetic link to any future child. You will finally move into an acceptance that, although this is not how you perceived it, the future carries the much-needed increased hope for a successful pregnancy. It can also be an opportunity to consider whether creating your family with donation support is for you or whether you feel more comfortable without donation.

It is important to note that some individuals and couples may feel ready to move forward with donation without experiencing deep feelings of grief or loss. They may have already had donation as a Plan B in their minds for quite some time and can proceed with treatment soon after an unsuccessful IVF treatment cycle. This is a very individual and couple-specific process.

Discussion about what donation means to you individually and as a couple, while also keeping in mind what it could mean for a potential child, can be daunting. It requires that you think about the future, taking into consideration your prospective needs and those of an adult donor child. This is difficult at a time when you are also trying to come to terms with your own loss around your dreams of having a child with biological connections to you.

Fertility counselling involves exploring these implications further. Many fertility clinics offer one implications counselling session for individuals and couples considering donation.

However, as it can include some complex issues to reflect on, many individuals and couples choose to have further exploratory fertility counselling to assist them in their decision-making process. This can include giving time to honour those feelings of loss and to gain some sense of closure before moving forward with any decision. It can also help to address any concerns about whether and how to disclose your decision to family members or close friends, and also to explore what disclosure or non-disclosure may mean to a potential child or future adult born from donation.

Implications counselling is recommended by the World Health Organization[8] and many of the governing authorities overseeing fertility clinics, such as the HFEA, ESHRE and ASRM. It will usually involve psycho-educational materials relating to donation as part of the therapeutic process, for example, further information regarding disclosure and, depending on the therapist, may include CBT resources to help you map out your decision-making process and reveal any in-depth beliefs or values that you may hold about each available option.

Unfortunately for many couples and individuals, these decisions are being made at a difficult time when they are also trying to consider how to increase the likelihood of having a pregnancy and all its associated considerations for treatment. It is difficult to consider how it may be for an adult donor child when you are trying to achieve a pregnancy! However, should you be successful, considering your options at this point will help your family in the future, long after fertility treatments are no longer part of your life.

As there is more research literature now available with regards to the experiences of adult donor children and their families, specific support organizations have been established to support decision making in this area. Such organizations aim to help families to effectively manage any issues or concerns regarding donation and disclosure by providing information, literature and support for before, during and after treatment (please see page 249 for more information).

## Who is it Recommended For?

Donation is recommended for the following reasons:

- You have a low egg reserve or compromised egg quality and have a very low percentage chance of conceiving without donation.
- You have a low sperm count or compromised sperm quality – morphology and motility – and have a very low percentage chance of conceiving without donation.
- You are a carrier of a genetic disease such as cystic fibrosis, which is considered likely to be passed on.
- You have had several unsuccessful IVF cycles.
- You are post-menopausal.
- You have undergone previous medical treatment, for example, chemotherapy, which has compromised egg or sperm availability.
- You are in a same-sex relationship and require sperm donation to have a child.
- You are in a same-sex relationship and as a couple have decided to have treatment using your partner's eggs.
- You are single and want to have a child.

Recipient Treatment Options

## 1. Egg Donation

Following a consultation with your fertility doctor, you will attend an egg donation coordinator (usually a nurse or specialist in this area) and they will coordinate and discuss your treatment plan. All donors and recipients undertake full medical screening and this includes blood tests for hepatitis B and C, HIV, human T-cell viruses and sexually transmitted infections. The usual treatment protocol requires that recipient individuals and couples will attend a consultation with the clinic's fertility consultant and egg donation coordinator in addition to attending implications counselling with a fertility counsellor.

The donor will also undertake their process of assessment, screening and treatment by fertility consultants, nurses and the fertility counsellor. This may happen within the same clinic or via an external donation agency working with your treating clinic.

Once you have been matched with a suitable donor, you will receive fertility medication to synchronize your menstrual cycle with your donor's (also taking fertility medication for IVF egg retrieval). This medication will also prepare the lining of your womb so that it is suitable for embryo transfer and implantation.

In advance of this, some clinics may request that you undertake an 'assessment cycle' to ensure that they are aware of any problems, for example with the uterus lining, that may need to be rectified, in advance of the 'live' synchronized treatment cycle.

Following egg retrieval, the donated eggs are fertilized with the prepared sperm (this may involve ICSI) in the laboratory and you will have embryo transfer of the best-graded viable embryos 3–5 days later (blastocyst stage occurs at Day 5 and it is common to transfer then). You will continue to take progesterone during the two-week wait period, to support embryo implantation and a continuation of pregnancy, should it be successful. You will discuss with your consultant in advance whether it will involve one or two embryo transfers.

## 2.  Sperm Donation

As outlined above, sperm donation may be recommended by your consultant if you have had several unsuccessful IVF cycles and sperm quantity or quality is a factor, or if you need it as a result of a previous medical procedure (for example, after cancer treatment or a vasectomy). Donated sperm is also used for single women and couples in same-sex relationships undergoing IUI or IVF treatment. The treatment approach recommended by your consultant is dependent on your presenting medical factors as an individual, and combined factors as a couple.

In general, licensed clinics will only work with sperm donation agencies that provide sperm to the quality standards outlined by the medical governing bodies for fertility clinics (for example, the HFEA, ESHRE, ASRM and WHO), in addition to quality standards for best practice, outlined by their own embryology department.

The donation banks screen donors to ensure that they are not carriers for infectious diseases such as HIV and hepatitis B and C. Donors are also screened for any sexual diseases during their health check. They will also undertake implications counselling (usually one session) before committing to becoming a donor.

Many women and couples undertake several cycles of IUI or IVF with sperm donation to increase the likelihood of success.

### Choosing your donor

There are limits on the number of children that can be created using a particular donor. This is dependent on the country you reside in. In most clinics (not all), you are responsible for ordering the sperm using an online ordering process. The donated sperm is then delivered to the laboratory in the treating clinic, using stringent quality transfer procedures. Most clinics support you in this process by providing you with a step-by-step guide on how to order the sperm.

Sperm banks usually offer 'identifiable' and 'anonymous' donor choices. There is also an option of choosing a 'basic' or 'extended' donor profile. In general, choosing an extended profile will provide you with more expansive information (for example, medical history for extended family of the donor), which you may find helpful in the present, and also which you may choose to pass on to your child/adult child in response to questions they may ask in the future.

Choosing an 'identifiable' or 'anonymous' donor presents other important factors for consideration. Following much consultation and research, some countries have changed their legislation with regards to fertility treatment clinics and no longer allow 'anonymous' donation (for example the UK and, most recently, Ireland). This means you will need to select a 'UK compliant' or 'identifiable' donor when you are choosing your sperm donor for treatment. If you are choosing to have treatment with an identifiable 'known' donor (for example a relative or friend), they will be required to undertake the same stringent medical and consultation procedures, as is required by donation agencies. This will happen in your treatment clinic.

**Journal Activity: Known Donation – points to consider** 🖊

- What does it mean for you to move forward with a known donor in treatment?
- What are your expectations in regards to your donor before, during and after treatment?
- If you have other children (secondary infertility problems), have you considered how to relay the information to them?
- What are your expectations (if any) in regards to any potential child and agreed contact/or not with the known donor?
- Has this understanding been communicated between you and the donor?
- Is your relationship with your donor solid enough to maintain these expectations now and in the future?
- Is your donor aware of the screening and medical procedures and time necessary to go through treatment?
- If your known donor is a relative, will you be letting other family members know of your treatment? Is the donor aware and in agreement with this?
- Will your donor be letting her/his children know?
- What may happen if your family know and you choose not to tell your child?
- What may happen if your family know and you choose to tell your child?

### Journal Activity: Considering Egg or Sperm Donation 🖊

As donation is a more complex treatment option to consider, it can be helpful to work through what it may mean to you individually and as a couple; on a psychological, emotional, physical, financial and perhaps social level.

Allow yourself plenty of time to reflect fully on what emerges for you, and as a couple, when completing each of the enquiry questions below:

* Do you feel that you have resolved, as best you can, the feelings of loss associated with letting go of your hope for a child genetically connected to you and your partner? Have you allowed yourself the space to process this?
* Do you feel that you and your partner are in agreement in regards to what it means to move forward with donation?
* What are your thoughts and feelings around this?
* What are your thoughts and feelings about the donor? Being open and positive about your choice to move forward with donation and accepting that a donor is part of this process is likely to support you in bonding with your pregnancy and your process of becoming a mother with the help of donation.
* Equally, if you have strong thoughts or feelings of resistance it may not be the treatment choice for you.

- Naturally it takes time to work through your feelings from grief and loss if IVF treatment does not work towards being open to donation or not. Write about this without stopping to edit or correct yourself. This journaling exercise may be one that you take some time to do. You can revisit it as often as you want until you have resolved it enough to make the decision.
- Are you considering anonymous/unknown or identifiable/unknown donation?
    - What are the benefits to you individually or as a couple in the short /long term in making this choice?
    - What are the costs to you individually or as a couple in the short /long term in making this choice?
    - What are the potential benefits to a donor child/ adult in making this choice in the short /long term?
    - What are the potential costs to a donor child/ adult in making this choice in the short /long term?
    - How might this be for them?
- Are you considering known donation?
    - What are the benefits in the short /long term in making this choice?
    - What are the costs in the short /long term in making this choice?

## Egg Sharing

If there is a significant male-factor problem, but no female-factor problem affecting egg quality or availability, some couples and individual women choose egg-sharing treatment. This option usually facilitates private fertility treatment, where the couple or individual woman donates eggs and can then choose to undergo treatment themselves as a couple for male-factor fertility problems, at a much reduced rate. Many women who decide on this treatment option perceive it as helping others (providing eggs via egg retrieval for recipient donor egg treatment) while also helping themselves (undertaking IVF treatment at a reduced rate). They can generally empathize with other couples undergoing fertility treatment as they require their own treatment, although for different reasons (not involving egg reserve/quality).

Journal Activity: Contemplating Egg Sharing: 🖉

* Are you aware of the medical procedures and risks involved?
* Are both you and your partner in agreement about your decision to donate eggs?
* How may you feel if it is successful for you and also a recipient individual/couple?
* How may you feel if it is unsuccessful for you and successful for a recipient individual/couple?

- If you already have a child, have you considered how you may explain your donation to your child, should it be successful for the recipient couple?
- Are you aware that an adult donor child may request contact or further information when they reach 18 or older?

## Managing the Two-week Wait

Whether you are following a natural cycle without medication or undergoing IUI, IVF or donor treatment, you will need to wait for two weeks to know if you have a positive pregnancy. Many patients describe this as the most challenging time of the treatment. Sitting with uncertainty is difficult for most people. However, this 'waiting' is following intense investment on all levels and naturally your whole being wants to know the answer – has it worked? You may oscillate between the certainty of knowing it has or has not, often within minutes of each other.

Naturally, overthinking will not impact on your chances. However, when we feel that something is out of our control, it is a natural instinct to endeavour to think our way around the situation. Mindfulness with self-compassion can help you to be more present to where you are now, and kindness and distraction techniques can support you to have some moments where the pregnancy result is not filling your every thought.

Research indicates that a combination of relaxation techniques and distraction has been shown to best support stress reduction during this period.[9]

## Stress-less Mindfulness

On a daily basis, or several times a day if you have the available time, alternate between the mindful check-in and body scan exercise in Chapter 2 (pages 27 and 57). You can combine this with the mindfulness exercise for loving-kindness in Chapter 8 (see page 205).

### Tips for Overthinking

Can you really trust your thoughts, when one moment they are telling you that you are definitely pregnant and the very next your busy mind is telling you that you can't be? Just notice these thoughts and give them a description. Draw on your ability to generate a more encouraging self-dialogue, for example:

> 'Noticing that I have busy "I am" and "am not" thoughts. They are just thoughts, not facts that I need to follow. I am saying "yes" to the possibility that I am pregnant and I have tried all that I can do to achieve a pregnancy. It is as it is right now and I can take care of myself with kindness. I care for and accept myself as I am now in this moment and send loving-kindness towards all of me.'

### Object of Attention

Do you have a favourite place that you visit or have visited that brings you a sense of inner happiness? You can elicit thoughts and memories of this place to generate a positive internal emotional experience. Having a picture that reminds you of this space can help you to begin to think about it and how it might feel to be there. Notice these feelings and the thoughts that accompany them. Of course, if your favourite place is somewhere close by or in your home you can take yourself there and become very present to the support it brings. You may wish to integrate the safe place exercise in Chapter 2 (page 62) to deepen this experience.

## Managing Family and Friends

Some people let everybody know that they are going through an assisted-fertility cycle to gain the emotional support that they need. Others limit the number of people they share this information with as it can otherwise mean daily updates to a large circle of people. Remember, the priority is to take care of yourself and you may decide that it is easier to let people know that they will hear from you in two weeks in a way that feels manageable for you, for example, via text if successful, and that if they do not hear from you to respect your space until you feel ready to contact them.

Decide with your partner how and where you will do the pregnancy test. It is important whether undertaking treatment in a relationship or not that you have a trusted and supportive individual to honour this important milestone with.

## Nurture Yourself

It is not always easy to take gentle care of yourself when you are feeling emotionally stressed. The chapter on self-care (page 189) will offer some self-caring ideas and distracting activities to draw on, to support you during this vulnerable time. You may wish to distract yourself with some uplifting movies that don't require much engagement or take some walks in nature to feel grounded. This time is about supporting, not challenging, yourself so perhaps limit the things you don't enjoy, for example, planning to have a friend or relative over who may ask intrusive questions will not help in distracting you, although a helpful friend who offers to cook and keep you company could be welcome! Be led by your needs.

## Noticing Physical Symptoms

Some women describe feeling pregnant and then not feeling the symptoms and subsequently make negative assumptions about this. The symptoms of nausea and tiredness can be attributed to early pregnancy or the progesterone you are taking. They can also be the physiological response to the psychological impact of this incredibly important event. Therefore, expect the symptoms to come and go and notice the sensations with self-kindness and without bringing judgement or evaluation to the varying pleasant or unpleasant sensations.

## Mini Relaxation Techniques

We often carry tension in our shoulders. Close your eyes and lift your shoulders up towards your ears as you breathe in for one, two, three. Hold your shoulders up for three seconds, then rotate them back and down slowly, releasing down on the out-breath for three seconds. I have discovered you can do this on a very busy train without attracting too much attention to yourself! In other words, mindfulness and relaxation techniques can be integrated into busy schedules or when awaiting an outcome, for example when sitting in the waiting room before seeing your medical practitioner.

The healing breath in Chapter 6 (page 145) and the three-minute mindful check-in (page 27) can also help to ground you in the present and restore a sense of internal balance beneath the busy planning mind.

## Do I Need to Take Extra Care of Myself?

It is usually advisable to resume normal day-to-day activities but to avoid strenuous, overexertion, for example finding gentle ways to reduce stress rather than engaging with high-impact exercise. The general guideline is to act as if you are pregnant – avoiding raw fish, synthetic sweeteners or cream cheese, etc., avoiding lifting heavy objects and staying away from highly stressful environments – but to not avoid normal day-to-day living and expectations.

## Moving on from Treatment

### A Positive Pregnancy Test

The excitement of seeing that faint pink line confirm the much-awaited positive pregnancy usually brings with it a flux of intense emotions. One woman expressed to me that she was so over-whelmed with emotion she began crying inconsolably until she realized that her husband had thought it was an unsuccessful cycle and began offering words of comfort. So, firstly, be sure to let your partner know the result!

Elated joy and an immense sense of relief can be followed by some anxiety – this is perfectly normal, especially if you have had assisted reproductive treatment. It is a good idea if attending a fertility clinic to arrange a follow-up pregnancy test to allay some of those fears. They will also track your pregnancy hormone levels.

Usually the care continues in a fertility clinic until 12 weeks into the pregnancy, as after this time the risk of miscarriage drops significantly to only 1 per cent. Part of the care will involve giving what is known as the 'pregnancy hormone' – progesterone supplementation – to support a healthy pregnancy. It is also commonly used as a preventative therapy for women who have experienced miscarriage in the past. Folic acid will also be prescribed due to its important role in cell production and division. The first trimester has some significant milestones, and women tend to experience a reduction in fear as each one passes. One such milestone – the seven-week scan – can be an exciting time as it is when you and your partner will hear your baby's heartbeat for the first time.

Whether you have achieved a pregnancy naturally or with assisted fertility treatment, it is a good idea to visit your GP and inform them of your pregnancy result and any relevant fertility medical treatment undertaken. They can then discuss your care options – this is important, especially if you have ever experienced a previous miscarriage. If this is the case, you may require very close monitored care or 'perinatology' – specialized care of women and pregnancy.

Having a proactive approach to your health can also help you during this time. Most women who have undertaken natural or assisted fertility treatment have considered their physical and emotional health, and it is important to continue to engage with stress reduction support and a nutritional and supplementation pregnancy care plan. There are many excellent books to help take you through the stages from early pregnancy to delivery with recommendations on dietary and lifestyle choices. They are usually accompanied by wonderful pictures of the developing foetus which will help you connect with the reality of your growing pregnancy.

As when undergoing assisted fertility treatment, gentle and restorative exercise is advised rather than anything high impact or overstrenuous for the body. There are plenty of pregnancy yoga classes that combine gentle poses with breathwork to benefit physical and emotional balance. Classes such as this can also allow you dedicated time towards establishing a deeper connection with your pregnancy.

## Mountain Meditation

I have worked with many women during the early stages of pregnancy who express feelings of guilt at not having the levels of joy they presumed they would have, combined with recurrent anxious thinking. It is not uncommon to feel out of sync with other pregnant women and even your partner, as the predominant feelings you experience fluctuate between stress, joy, numbness and disbelief. Expressing these feelings and also supporting any necessary change in beliefs or thinking patterns, combined with stress reduction skills, can help to ease you into feelings of self-compassion, calming your mind and encouraging a gentle bonding process to begin.

Try the following 'mountain meditation' to help you calm the mind and feel grounded within. Mountains are usually majestic and evoke an image of strength and endurance. They represent a good metaphor to draw from. Connecting with a mountain visualization can help you to regain your own inner strength and to feel reconnected with your deeper self and your growing baby within.

- Sit in a comfortable, upright and dignified posture with the soles of your feet connecting to the ground beneath.
- Begin taking some deep mindful breaths, growing more connected and present with each inhale and exhale. Take a deep breath in through your nostrils and release slowly on the out-breath, with your mouth slightly open and shaped in a loose circle.
- Now as you breathe in through your nose, expand your area of focus to include your whole body. Follow your full

inhale and exhale of breath as it enters and leaves your body. Soften your attention and allow all of the sensations – pleasant and unpleasant – to flow, enveloping them in an open and non-judgemental way.

- Imagine that you are sitting facing a mountain in the near distance. This may be a mountain that you have visited or one that you have seen an image of.

- Visualize this mountain and appreciate its grandness of scale, noticing how solid it sits even if the winds of change blow. Examine the detail of this mountain more closely; its rocky edges and grassy verges. Notice whether it is a lush green or a charcoal grey. Take in all the detail that defines its strong presence.

- Let this mountain inspire you to connect with the strength you also carry within. Consider all the strength you have needed to take you to where you are today.

- Now rest your awareness on your inner world – what thoughts are passing through your mind? Can you notice these thoughts as just mental activity, as though clouds passing above the mountain top? Allow the thoughts to pass without trying to change or hold them.

- Following on from this, gently ease your focus of attention on to the sensations within and where you store them in your body. Notice any areas of tension or resistance. Allow the changing feelings and sensations to be present and, like the mountain, accept these ever-changing landscapes while remaining strong in the vastness of your true self.

- Let your breath anchor you to your unshakeable strength and steadiness within. Notice the stillness deepen with each in-breath and release any feelings of fear by letting go on each out-breath.

- Feel the harmony of your mind and body as it connects to the earth beneath. As you close this meditation, repeat the phrase: 'I am strong, I am grounded and I am present to this "now" moment.'

- Feel your connectedness expand to your heart, body and your growing baby within. May you continue to grow in strength together. 'I am here, we are here, we grow strong together.'

### If Treatment is Unsuccessful

If the pregnancy test is negative, it is likely to give rise to many questions in addition to feelings of disillusionment and loss. Allowing the time to express these strong feelings before moving on to any Plan B is important to honour the process you have just invested so much in. Chapter 1 takes you through the stages of grief and loss often associated with an unsuccessful treatment cycle or biochemical pregnancy. This process can include: shock, protest or denial, bargaining, anger, depression, testing and acceptance. Take time and space to process these feelings, as being mindful of our emotions also allows us to move through them rather than numbing out and making reactive decisions we may later regret. Loving-kindness meditation (page 205) and also journaling to heal (page 47) can help you to move consciously through your feelings, thoughts and sensations with a deeper awareness.

It is important to book back in to see your consultant if you have undertaken assisted fertility treatment. An unsuccessful cycle carries learning as well as loss, and the consultant may have further information to consider, having reviewed all the stages of the treatment and its unfortunate outcome. This may include information relating to your ovarian response, egg or sperm quality, or observations about embryo development or the womb lining.

The consultant may recommend a different protocol or another type of treatment for you to consider. Being prepared for this return consultation can facilitate you in making a decision about whether you want to consider another treatment option or to face an end of treatment. The decision to end treatment is naturally a difficult one and it will be helped if it is informed by what the likely reasons are for your treatment having not worked. If you decide to continue with treatment, the return consultation can help to consolidate your treatment options.

The following questions are important to keep in mind for your follow-up consultation:

- What are the likely reasons that your treatment did not work?
- What are your options (treatment and non-treatment) moving forward?
- How likely is it for a new treatment option to work?

Should you decide as an individual or a couple that the wisest choice present is to end treatment, it is important to acknowledge to yourselves that you and your consultant have given it your best. Sometimes ending treatment is giving yourself the best care you can at that time. It is the treatment that has been unsuccessful, not that you have failed – there is an important difference and this is often overlooked!

It is likely that you have reached this decision for a variety of reasons – it is emotionally, psychologically or financially too wearing to continue and you understand that not every couple will have a baby with fertility treatment. It is wise to write down your decision-making process so that you can remind yourself of your informed decision in times of doubt or sadness. You may decide to move forward and, after a time caring for yourself as individuals and as a couple, consider focusing on other areas of your life and relationship without fertility treatment. Some couples after a time of reflection and healing explore the option of having a child with adoption.

I believe that taking an integrative approach to your health-care gives you the best chance at conceiving, as a healthy body supports a healthy mind and vice versa. Complementary therapies are generally integrated as a way of life and can therefore benefit your health during natural, assisted or integrated treatment and beyond. The following chapter explores various natural therapies in detail.

# CHAPTER 4

## *Natural Health Therapies*

We have all experienced feeling out of internal balance, either through busy lives or as a result of health issues, and natural therapies can help individuals to restore a sense of harmony to their mind and body. Natural health therapy has been used for centuries to relieve symptoms and promote good health; acupuncture needles have been unearthed in archaeological sites in China that date back to the Shang dynasty (1500BC) and nowadays hospitals throughout China routinely combine modern Western medicine with traditional Chinese medicine to treat illness and promote optimum health. Rather than taking an 'either/or' approach, complementary medicine can feel more in keeping with your life choices, whatever fertility health system you are engaged with. In the right hands holistic health is generally safe and can support you in making the lifestyle and health changes necessary to enhance your chances of a positive pregnancy, while also helping to support your emotional and psychological health. There is a reason these therapies have stood the test of time.

The main natural health therapies are outlined below. Take some time to think about which treatments would best support your personal health and well-being, and support you in achieving your fertility goals. Please bear in mind that, like any healthcare system, there are alternative therapies that can promote health and well-being and others that only claim to do so. Therefore finding the right therapist can be as important as the therapy you choose. Be mindful of any therapy or practitioner that offers a miracle cure for fertility.

## Acupuncture

Acupuncture has a long tradition of being used to support fertility problems. However, its popularity as an adjunct therapy to mainstream medical fertility treatment increased following a publication by the World Health Organization in 2002 citing the benefits of acupuncture for some fertility-related problems.[1]

Further research found that when 80 of 160 women undertaking IVF with 'good quality' embryos received acupuncture before and after embryo implantation, success rates reported after six weeks were 42.3 per cent compared with 26.3 per cent in the 80 women who received no acupuncture.[2] While there is an abundance of more recent research relating to the health benefits of acupuncture combined with Traditional Chinese

Medicine (TCM), these specific reports prompted the increase of acupuncture being used in conjunction with Western medicine for fertility-related problems. Further studies have also stated that acupuncture before and after embryo transfer increases pregnancy outcomes for women undertaking IVF.[3] In general, acupuncture is used to support men and women throughout the IVF process and not just pre- and post-embryo transfer. It is thought to support optimum endometrium conditions and overall fertility health.[4]

More recent research claimed a 65 per cent improvement in IVF outcomes when combined with acupuncture.[5] However, the National Health Service (NHS) in the UK, which funds acupuncture for some forms of pain relief, has stated that further research would be required into these preliminary findings and cited several limitations in regards to this research.[6]

Overall, acupuncture is considered to be a safe natural health therapy: 'no clear trend in the frequency of reports of acupuncture related adverse events over the past 30 years.'[7] That being said, it is very important to attend a qualified and registered practitioner who practises acupuncture safely and only uses herbs that meet with quality control standards within the country of practice.

## What is Acupuncture?

Acupuncture uses very fine needles placed on points on the body known as 'meridians'. It is predominantly used in conjunction with TCM which also includes the use of herbs, and sometimes nutritional advice and exercise, for example tai chi or qigong and massage to promote good health.

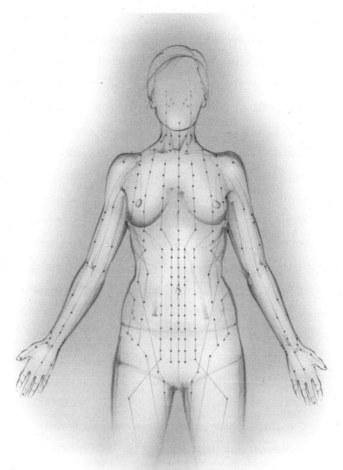

The main acupuncture meridian channels

Within TCM, it is believed that health is compromised when there is a stagnation of energy within the body causing one's body or mind to be out of balance. Acupuncture serves to balance this energy or 'chi' throughout the body. Traditional Chinese Medicine practitioners also pay close attention to the body's temperature and harmonizing the energy lines which they believe may be excessively yin (excessive heat in the system and kidneys) or yang (excessive cold and damp in the system). This is then linked to specific organs either over- or under-functioning, for example, affecting heart rate, blood flow, hormone balance, body temperature, energy levels and inflammation within the body and causing mood imbalance – anger, anxiety, sadness or a general feeling of being overwhelmed by emotions.

According to TCM, there are 12 main meridians and each one has a specific function or relates to a particular organ in the body. Assessment by a practitioner will include a full medical history and they will look for outward signs of internal imbalance by examining your complexion, taking your pulse and checking the texture, size and colour of your tongue. In their assessment, they will ask in-depth questions relating to your normal body temperature, your appetite and your sleeping patterns. They then treat any perceived imbalances with acupuncture by inserting very fine needles into the skin at meridian points or alternatively applying pressure to these points with acupressure. This is usually combined with dietary advice and sometimes herbal formulas.

## Choosing an Acupuncturist

Acupuncturists can train to specialize at Master's and PhD level and there is specific training received that relates to the protocols for fertility. In Switzerland, acupuncturists and herbalists (TCM approach) are also qualified GPs; countries in Europe and states within the US legislate differently. Legislation may include expanding or limiting requirements for the use of herbs with acupuncture practice. When choosing a therapist, it is important to ensure that they have also trained in the specialized area of fertility support. It is also beneficial if your practitioner has experience of working alongside patients receiving assisted reproductive medicine and treatment.

Sometimes medical practitioners can be overcautious about integrating natural-health therapies with mainstream treatment and, similarly, some natural health practitioners can be overcautious about a client's need to refer to a medical practitioner. When you take an integrative approach to your healthcare, it is most important to draw on the strengths of both the medical and natural healthcare systems to best support your overall health, healing and well-being. Unfortunately, working with many fertility patients, I have heard several claims made which are not helpful to a person's medical treatment or natural healthcare approach, for example, nobody can state that they can definitely make you pregnant within three months and equally no one can claim that you have some energy block to pregnancy. These invalidated claims are usually expressed to vulnerable people in an effort to secure a return visit and unfortunately they can impact severely on an individual's self-belief, triggering the person to over-personalize their level of responsibility – there is no such thing as a badly behaved ovary and you cannot unblock a fallopian tube with visualization!

Consider placing the qualities of 'integrity', 'reputation' and 'experience' at the top of your list when choosing a fertility health practitioner and this will support you on your fertility journey. Word-of-mouth recommendations are also helpful when making your choice and it is important to give appropriate consideration to the training and accreditation of practitioners. Finally, but not in order of importance, having a rapport with your treating healthcare practitioner will help to create a safe space for you to feel comfortable and trust in the care you are receiving.

An acupuncturist will aim to support fertility in the following ways:

- To stimulate the body's natural healing system.
- To increase blood flow to the uterus.
- To support a balance in the 'Vessel of Conception', by applying acupuncture to support functioning in the pituitary, thyroid, pancreas and uterus regions.
- To help regulate hormone balance.
- To accompany pre- and post-embryo transfer.
- To support quality and quantity of sperm when combined with lifestyle changes.
- To provide emotional support.

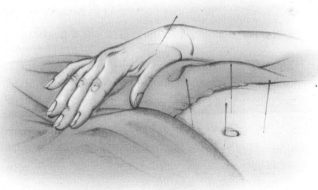

Acupuncturists work with specific protocols for
fertility support and stress reduction

The majority of fertility clinics do not recommend using herbs as part of an integrated healthcare approach when the individual is undergoing an IVF/IUI cycle. The concern is that the herbs could interact with the prescription drugs being taken in treatment. It is therefore important to consult with your treating doctor and natural-health practitioner to ensure that there are no contra-indications and follow their advice on whether or not to begin a course of herbal medicine with your acupuncture. Many patients undertaking more than one fertility treatment cycle opt for taking the herbs in between treatments. Herbs and acupuncture are usually used with nutritional therapy in the treatment of PCOS or endometriosis.

## Aromatherapy

We often live our lives connecting to our surroundings from our evaluating, thinking, and often judgemental, self: 'I like this . . .', 'I don't like this . . .', 'Why do this . . . ?' This stimulates us to move towards one experience and move away from others. This is our natural survival instinct at work, which is important for our welfare. However, it can sometimes dominate and as a result we disconnect from our intuitive, creative or felt sense. This is particularly true when experiencing fertility treatment where we tend to get caught in our planning mind. It can be helpful to reconnect to our environment through our sense of smell or touch. Aromatherapy can be beneficial for emotional well-being by relaxing the senses and thus improving mood.

Essential oils are extracted from plants – flowers, herbs or trees – and can be added to your bath (four drops is enough), used in massage 'carrier' oils, or in an aromatherapy oil burner (a few drops of oil are added to water and the candle beneath releases the aromas into the surrounding atmosphere).

As with most natural health therapies, aromatherapy has been around for many centuries, dating back to Egyptian times when it was used for medicinal purposes and in the mummification process! The phrase 'aromatherapy' became popular following the publication in 1937 of *Aromathérapie: Les Huiles Essentielles Hormones Végétales* by the French perfumer and chemist, René-Maurice Gattefossé.[8]

As many oils are combined in the use of aromatherapy massage, it is important to ensure that your massage therapist is fully trained in the use of aromatherapy oils. Oils are generally combined to elevate mood, for example, orange or mandarin oil to uplift the mood and lavender oil to relax the mind and promote restful sleep. In general, essential oils are used to energize, de-stress and promote well-being and relaxation.

Top Ten Essential Oils to Support Fertility Health and Help Reduce Stress:

1. Chamomile: relieves stress and anxiety and promotes better sleep. It is also anti-inflammatory (if used in massage).
2. Clary sage: relieves cramping if used in massage after egg collection. It is also relaxing and helps to reduce stress.
3. Fennel: aids digestion and is traditionally used to help with menstrual irregularities.
4. Frankincense: supports the immune system.

5. Ylang Ylang: traditionally used as an antidepressant and is also thought to be an aphrodisiac in addition to having sedative properties.
6. Geranium: traditionally used to support hormonal balance.
7. Lavender: promotes restful sleep and reduces stress.
8. Lemon: detoxes and uplifts the mood.
9. Neroli: elevates mood and reduces anxiety.
10. Peppermint: reduces nausea (can be used after egg collection as peppermint tea), relieves muscular pain and reduces migraines. Also has energizing properties.

It is important to only use combination oils in massage carrier oils with a qualified aromatherapy massage therapist or aromatherapist. You can use the above oils in oil burners and add them to your bath (maximum four drops per bath). You can also buy combinations in organic massage carrier oils in good health stores. Also, for quality assurance, it is advisable to buy organic essential oils.

## Naturopathy

Naturopathy draws on the healing abilities within nature to support a cure: the naturopath believes in the innate ability of nature to heal physical or emotional problems. Naturopathy became a popular way to treat and prevent illness in Germany in the 19th century, where it accompanied spa treatments for health promotion properties. In naturopathy the person is viewed in the whole or holistic sense. An initial assessment will consider the individual's physical, emotional and environmental influences. The practitioner will recommend health-promoting supplements and also natural herbal remedies for fertility support. However, remember to consult with your doctor before taking any herbs in conjunction with assisted reproductive treatment, for example IVF or IUI, due to possible interactions of medicine and herbs. The use of herbs is usually not recommended by clinicians during a cycle (see page 119).

Naturopaths will also provide information on the healing properties of foods and will make very specific dietary recommendations. Treatment plans will usually include an element of detoxification. The belief is that modern toxins and lifestyle habits impact negatively on psychological and physical health. Detoxification usually includes drinking specific quantities of water daily, and taking cleansing herbs and supplements. It may also include liver cleansing. (As with herbs, consult with your doctor before undertaking a detoxification programme.) A naturopath will also recommend foods and supplements to reduce inflammation, for example anti-candida foods, etc. This can be beneficial following treatment for endometriosis.

A naturopath will focus on strengthening the immune system with herbs, supplements and eliminating processed foods from the diet. They may also assess for food allergies or sensitivities. Some naturopaths use some animal-based hormones for use as thyroid supplements. This may not be appropriate if you are currently attending a fertility clinic. Please check with your consultant first before taking.

Naturopathy is regarded as a preventative approach to healthcare and the information received is to support the individual in becoming more proactive in the management of their own health and self-care.

## Biodynamic Massage

Biodynamic massage is a form of massage that aims to provide healing on a mind and body level. It was first established in the 1960s by Gerda Boyesen, a psychologist who was interested in the power of healing touch, especially where individuals have experienced physical or emotional distress.[9] Biodynamic massage works on the principle that physiological touch has an impact on neurological processes. The belief is that emotional processes are stored not just in the mind but also in the body.

Biodynamic massage is either used by holistic massage therapists specifically trained in the technique, or as part of a form of body psychotherapy, which explores the physiological effects of distress and aims to treat this on a psychological and physiological level. As with any form of therapy, it may appeal to some and not others. Some individuals may prefer to attend a psychotherapist for mind health and a massage therapist for body health, while others may find that biodynamic massage provides them with a space for deeper healing due to its integrated levels.

Biodynamic massage shares many of the same theoretical beliefs that are present within Ayurvedic massage and Shiatsu acupressure massage, namely the idea that the body is a vessel for emotional calm or distress, and this is manifest in energy blocks within the body. Healing massage is aimed at establishing a free energy flow within the body. For example, a person with very low mood may not feel physically connected but rather have a feeling of disconnect, or a stressed individual may become very busy but be unaware of the feelings within their body. There is then a potential for illness or disharmony to manifest without the awareness of the individual, for example, they could suffer from chronic fatigue without experiencing the onset of symptoms until they are unmanageable. Balance is restored to mind and body with the power of touch in a healing and supportive environment.

Past and present events can impact on what we 'hold' in our bodies and physiological healing may be required to encourage the person to feel more embodied. Just as pleasant memories can trigger pleasant physical sensations, so too our body responds to unpleasant memories. For example, entering a clinical setting may mean that you experience tightness in your chest and a tense jaw or shoulder muscles. This is probably based on a previous rather than present experience of your visit to the clinic. By bringing healing to this very physical memory, the biodynamic therapist aims to bring harmony back to mind and body.

Other benefits of biodynamic massage include:

- Tailoring the massage to the individual needs of the person and their presenting issues – physical or emotional.
- Where biodynamic massage is part of a body psychotherapy any previous body trauma will also be explored to concentrate the therapist on the areas requiring further attention. This can be beneficial to women who have felt a sense of disconnect after experiencing the

trauma of miscarriage, or if they have had several cycles of IVF and need some physiological healing after self-administering injections, etc.

Biodynamic massage can be experienced by attending a complementary therapist who is also specifically trained in this technique or a body psychotherapist specially trained in working with distress on a psychological level and how it manifests on a somatic level in our body.

As Hippocrates expressed wisely, 'Let food be thy medicine and medicine be thy food.' The following chapter by Dr Marilyn Glenville expands on how this can apply to enhancing your fertility health.

# CHAPTER 5

## *Using Nutrition and Supplements to Boost Fertility by Dr Marilyn Glenville*

*Dr Marilyn Glenville is one of the UK's leading nutritionists, specializing in women's health. She is the former President of the Food and Health Forum at the Royal Society of Medicine and brings a wealth of expertise on how to optimize fertility health with dietary improvements and supplements. What we take into our body can positively influence our fertility health, as outlined in this chapter by Dr Glenville.*

Fertility is dependent on a number of factors, so diet, lifestyle, environmental toxins and emotional issues are all important for improving natural conception, reducing the risk of miscarriage and enhancing the success rate of an IVF cycle or any assisted conception technique.

More and more women are having babies later in life. In 2013 the number of births to mothers aged 25–34 was more than double the number to mothers aged under 25. However, in between 1967 and 1971 births to mothers aged under 25 exceeded births to mothers aged 25–34.[1]

The average age of all mothers giving birth is now 31; the highest ever. But even though 40 is becoming the new 30 (or 20 even) and women are living longer and feeling and looking younger, the undeniable truth is that the biological clock still ticks away at the same rate it did a generation ago, and a woman is still considered to be in her reproductive prime in her twenties. Past the age of 35 the clock speeds up making it more difficult to conceive, even if you are trying for your second or third child.

For many years it was thought that age only mattered with women when it came to fertility but we now know that the man's age counts too. Men do have a biological clock and, like women's, it decreases more rapidly over the age of 35. Research has shown that with men over the age of 35 the sperm count can be lower and the sperm are less motile, and the risk of miscarriage is increased in women whose partners are over 35.[2] Some men may be on their second relationship having already had children, but because they are older they may be finding it more difficult to conceive.

As a woman the amount of eggs (your ovarian reserve) is set and can't be altered because the store was established in your body since before you were born. Most women are born with about 2 million egg follicles; by puberty there are about 750,000; and by the age of around 45, as few as 10,000 may be left. If you are going for an assisted-conception technique, like IUI, IVF or ICSI, you will also want to be as healthy as possible to give the technique the best chance. With a national average success rate in the UK for IVF of between 20 and 32 per cent for women under the age of 40, it is important to do whatever you can to improve your health, which can be supported by improving your nutrition and lifestyle.[3]

## Causes of Infertility

We know that infertility can be caused by a number of medical problems including:

| | |
|---|---|
| Ovulatory failure (including PCOS) | 20% |
| Tubal damage | 15% |
| Endometriosis | 5% |
| Male problems | 26% |
| Unexplained | 30% |
| Other | 4% |

Many couples can experience more than one problem when trying to conceive: for example, the woman may suffer from endometriosis, but her partner may also have a low sperm count.

'Unexplained' is the most common diagnosis for infertility which unfortunately just means that there is no diagnosed medical reason why you are not getting pregnant. There may, of course, be another reason which can include not only looking at your diet and checking for nutritional deficiencies, but also thinking about lifestyle and emotional issues.

Usually doctors will consider a diagnosis of infertility after at least a year has passed.

## Three Months' Pre-conception Care

Three months is the magic number to really concentrate on integrating a healthy dietary plan and improving other lifestyle areas. It can be helpful to seek support from a nutritionist who specializes in the area of fertility as they are likely to recommend dietary changes and supplements specific to your individual needs.

Many women have high FSH or low AMH levels, indicating lower ovarian reserve, and this makes it difficult for their bodies to respond to the IVF drugs, but it does not stop them conceiving naturally albeit with a lower chance of conception and it makes sense to be at your optimum health to support a positive outcome.

With men, it takes at least three months for a new batch of sperm cells to mature, ready to be ejaculated. Men produce sperm all their lives so it is usually possible not only to improve the quality but also the quantity with lifestyle and nutritional changes.

**Diet**

Although it goes without saying that a healthy diet is crucial to a successful pregnancy and a healthy baby, many people are unaware of the fact that diet can help to correct hormone imbalances and other fertility issues that may affect your ability to conceive.[4] The following should be included in your diet:

- Plenty of fruit and vegetables.
- Complex carbohydrates – wholegrains like brown rice, oats and wholemeal bread.

- Organic foods where possible.
- Oily foods such as fish, nuts, seeds and oils.
- Reduced intake of saturated fats from dairy products.
- Increased intake of fibre.
- Avoid additives, preservatives and chemicals, such as artificial sweeteners.
- Avoid sugar, both on its own and hidden in food.

Eating the right type of fats is particularly important for fertility. Just small increases in the consumption of trans fats can double the risk of anovulatory infertility. Also for problems with ovulation like PCOS, substituting just 5 per cent of your calorie intake as vegetable protein rather than animal protein reduces the risk of not ovulating by 50 per cent.[5]

Having four cups of coffee or any caffeinated drink a day makes it 26 per cent less likely that you will conceive[6] and drinking only two cups of coffee (200mg of caffeine) a day is associated with a 25 per cent increased risk of miscarriage.[7] Problems with sperm health are also connected with increased coffee intake.[8]

Alcohol will also make it more difficult for you to get pregnant[9] and that applies to the man too. Alcohol can lower sperm counts and will also block the body's ability to absorb fertility-boosting nutrients, such as zinc. Alcohol can also cause abnormalities in the head of the sperm which is important for healthy fertilization.[10]

## Lifestyle

A woman is twice as likely to get pregnant if she doesn't smoke compared to a woman who does.[11] And smoking is linked to 5,000 miscarriages per year.[12]

Stopping smoking is just as important for men. We know that chemicals in tobacco smoke can damage DNA in sperm, which can make it harder to conceive because fertilization can't take place or, if it is does, it can increase the risk of a miscarriage as nature will always work on survival of the fittest. Smoking can also affect sperm count, motility and the morphology (the shape of the sperm), whereby it could have two heads or two tails if the morphology is abnormal. Smoking also has a negative effect on the head of the sperm making it harder to fertilize an egg. It is thought that nicotine overloads the receptors on sperm, affecting their ability to bind to the egg.[13]

Smoking also reduces the chances of an IVF treatment being successful. If couples smoke during the IVF cycle the number of eggs retrieved is decreased by 40 per cent, and 46 per cent if just the man smokes during the cycle. Also, the overall success rate of the IVF is 44 per cent for non-smokers and 24 per cent for smokers.[14]

Other simple lifestyle changes for the man can include avoiding hot baths and tight underpants as sperm production takes place at 32°C (89°F) which is lower than the body temperature of 37°C (98.4°F). The testes are on the outside of a man's body to keep them cooler, but if they get too close to the body, for example, by sitting for long periods when driving, the sperm can heat up and reduce the count.

Men using laptops on their laps is also a problem for sperm health. In order to balance the laptop, men will often close their legs and this on its own (even without the laptop) raises the temperature of their genitals by up to 2.1°C. But the laptop itself generates heat and the combination of closing the legs and the heat from the laptop causes a rise in temperature of up to 2.8°C. Just a rise of 1°C can decrease fertility by 40 per cent.[15]

It's worth noting that if a couple has a combination of four negative lifestyle factors (including tea/coffee, smoking and alcohol) it can take them seven times longer to get pregnant.[16]

## Fertility-boosting Supplements

As well as looking at what you eat and drink there is now a great deal of scientific knowledge about the use of nutritional supplements and their beneficial effects on boosting fertility. We know that certain nutrients increase the chances of getting pregnant and staying pregnant either for natural conception or alongside IVF.

### Folic Acid

It is well known that folic acid can prevent spina bifida. Folic acid is undoubtedly important, but it is just part of the very important B-complex family of vitamins that are necessary to produce the genetic materials DNA and RNA.

### Zinc

Zinc is the most widely studied nutrient in terms of fertility for both men and women. It is an essential component of genetic material and a zinc deficiency can cause chromosome changes in either men or women, leading to reduced fertility and an increased risk of miscarriage. Zinc is found in high concentrations in the sperm and is needed to make the outer layer and tail of the sperm and is therefore essential for the health of sperm. To show you how powerful these nutrients are, men who were subfertile were given a combination of zinc and folic acid and they showed a 74 per cent increase in total sperm count.[17]

### Selenium

Selenium is an antioxidant that helps to protect your body from highly reactive chemical fragments called free radicals. For this reason, selenium can prevent chromosome breakage, which is known to be a cause of birth defects and miscarriages. Good levels of selenium are also essential to maximize sperm formation. Selenium supplementation given to infertile men increased sperm count, motility and the number of normal sperm.[18]

### Vitamin E

Vitamin E is another powerful antioxidant and has been shown to increase fertility when given to both men and women. With men, vitamin E helps to increase fertilization rates during ICSI treatments.[19] If a woman over the age of 35 is told that her fertility problems are caused by her age, then it is likely that she could benefit from taking both vitamins E and C.[20]

### Vitamin C

Vitamin C is also an antioxidant and we know that women with an increased intake of vitamin C (and a BMI under 25) have a shorter time to pregnancy. Vitamin C is also good for men as it can help to increase sperm counts by up to a third.[21]

Antioxidants in general (and these include zinc, selenium, vitamin C and vitamin E) have been shown to have a major impact on male fertility. A review of 34 studies with men going for IVF/ICSI cycles has shown that when men take antioxidants their partner is five times more likely to have a live birth compared to when taking a placebo.[22]

### Amino Acids

Two amino acids, L-arginine and L-carnitine, are particularly important for male fertility. L-arginine is essential for healthy sperm production and protects the sperm against oxidative damage.[23] The higher the levels of L-carnitine in sperm cells, the higher the sperm count and motility.[24]

### Omega-3 Fatty Acids

Omega-3 fatty acids have far-reaching effects for both male and female fertility. Sometimes immune problems may be affecting a woman's ability to get and stay pregnant. The theory is that in order for her body to stay pregnant, her immune system has to quieten down because half the baby's DNA is not hers. Normally if the body detects something foreign it aims to reject it and expel it from the body. For some women, their immune systems do not quieten down and so they can't get or stay pregnant.

One of the immune antibodies measured is called antiphospholipid antibodies (APAs). These blood-clotting antibodies can prevent implantation and cause recurrent miscarriage by attacking the cells that build the placenta. The medical treatment for this is blood thinners like aspirin and heparin. But research has shown that fish oil given to 22 women with APAs who already had three or more miscarriages went on to have 23 pregnancies (one woman had two babies during the study time frame) without a further miscarriage.[25] Omega-3 fatty acids are also important for male fertility because semen is rich in prostaglandins, which are produced from these omega-3 fatty acids. Men with poor sperm quality, abnormal sperm, poor motility or low count, can have inadequate levels of these beneficial prostaglandins and by supplementing with omega-3 fish oils there was a significant increase in sperm count compared to when taking a placebo.[26]

### Vitamin D

Vitamin D helps to regulate your immune system which, as we have seen with omega-3, is important in getting and staying pregnant. Vitamin D stops your immune system from over-reacting to the 'foreign' DNA from your partner in order to allow you to conceive and maintain that pregnancy.[27] Studies have shown that by deliberately making mice deficient in vitamin D they can actually become infertile.[28] Vitamin D is also important for male fertility as low levels of this nutrient are associated with low sperm motility and more abnormal forms.[29]

You manufacture vitamin D through your skin from the exposure to sunlight. But unfortunately more than half of adults in the UK have insufficient vitamin D levels.[30] Those most at risk in the UK are those who do not go out much in the daytime, those who do not expose their skin to the sunlight and women who wear make-up or cosmetics with in-built sun-protection factors.

We don't get much vitamin D from our food as our body expects us to manufacture it through our skin from the exposure to sunlight. It is found in oily fish, eggs and fortified breakfast cereals.

## Co-enzyme Q10

Your cells use this nutrient to produce energy and it also has antioxidant benefits. It has been studied extensively for male fertility and particularly for sperm motility as it is concentrated in the mitochondrial mid-piece of the sperm and provides energy for movement. Research shows that it not only helps with improving motility but can also increase sperm count and the number of normally formed sperm.[31]

It is only recently that it has been thought that co-enzyme Q10 might also be useful for women who are trying to conceive. It has been suggested that lower mitochondrial energy production may be at the root of 'ageing' eggs and co-enzyme Q10 is the fuel for the mitochondria, the powerhouses in your cells. One study showed that giving 'old' mice co-enzyme Q10 before ovarian stimulation improved not only egg quality but the number of eggs produced.[32]

## Stress and Fertility

You will have read in this book how important stress management is when you are aiming to get pregnant because too much stress can negatively affect the functioning of your pituitary gland which gives the message to your ovaries to release an egg at ovulation. The stress hormones also interfere with your production of progesterone which is the hormone that maintains the pregnancy for the first 12 weeks. So stress can make it harder to get pregnant and also to stay pregnant.

For women stress can also cause more testosterone to be produced and can lead to male symptoms such as hair growth (hirsutism), weight gain, acne and irregular menstrual cycles, and lead to PCOS.

Stress can also affect a man's fertility and even reduce sperm counts or increase the number of abnormal sperm. Stress can also affect sex drive for both you and your partner, and it is important that you have enough sex in order to give yourselves the best chance of conceiving.

### Controlling Your Blood Sugar

Balancing blood sugar is essential in lowering stress because the crashes in sugar levels which happen through the day (due to going long periods without food and not eating the right foods) stimulates more of the stress hormones. This is because these stress hormones, apart from helping you to run away from a tiger, can also mobilize your glucose (which has been stored as glycogen in the liver) back into the bloodstream. This is why you can feel more jittery, irritable, etc. when your blood sugar plummets!

To reduce your stress hormones nutritionally make sure you:

- Eat every three hours.
- Include some protein every time you eat, for example fish, eggs, quinoa, tofu, beans, nuts and seeds, and natural bio yoghurt. This slows down the release of sugar and thus keeps blood sugar levels more stable.
- Limit caffeine to one cup or avoid it if you can and never drink caffeine on an empty stomach because it is a stimulant and gets straight into the bloodstream and triggers cortisol release.
- Eat a serving of dark green leafy vegetables/salad daily.
- Snack on dried fruit (organic) and unsalted nuts and seeds.
- Replace white rice and bread with brown and wholemeal for fibre content and B vitamins.

## Important Nutrients for Reducing Stress

As well doing the best you can to control the release of the stress hormones from your pattern of eating, certain nutrients can be helpful. B vitamins (which are known as the 'stress' vitamins) are particularly useful in smoothing out the body's stress response, as are chromium to help with blood-sugar swings and magnesium, which is known as 'nature's tranquillizer'. These should all be in good levels in your fertility multivitamin and mineral so you do not need to take extra.

I know making these changes requires an effort on the couple's part but as research in the journal *Andrologia* in 2010 stated,

'There is strong evidence that complementary treatment with an appropriate nutraceutical improves the natural conception rate of infertile couples and increases the success rate of assisted reproductive techniques. Combating obesity, correcting inappropriate diet and banning the abuse of tobacco and alcohol are part of the integrated approach.'[34]

### Top Ten Fertility-boosting Tips

1.  Eat a diet rich in essential fats, from oily fish such as mackerel, sardines, wild salmon, pilchards and herring, to nuts and seeds. They are good for all body cells and can be used to manufacture and balance female hormones.

2.  Incorporate vitamin E rich foods which help to improve the quality and integrity of the zona pellucida (egg shell), which can harden and become more difficult for the sperm to penetrate. This gets harder with age, especially over the age of 35. Foods rich in vitamin E include seeds, almonds, hazelnuts and cashews.

3.  Zinc is essential for the quality of your eggs as it is an important antioxidant which protects the egg DNA. Foods rich in zinc include prawns and oysters, wheat germ, oats, corn, pumpkin, sunflower and sesame seeds, almonds, pecans, walnuts and Brazil nuts.

4.  Cut back on alcohol as this will affect your egg quality. In fact, drinking any alcohol at all can reduce your fertility by half – and the more you drink, the less likely you are to conceive.

5. Caffeine, particularly in the form of coffee, decreases fertility. Drinking as little as one cup of coffee a day can halve your chances of conceiving.

6. When you are trying to conceive, one of the most important things you need to do is to balance your hormones. Therefore minimize your exposure to 'xenoestrogens' which are essentially environmental oestrogens, coming from pesticides and the plastic industry and found in some cosmetics.

7. Avoid smoking as this has definitely been linked with infertility and can even bring on an early menopause, which is a particularly important consideration for older women who may be trying to beat the clock.

8. Manage stress by reviewing your work/life balance and learn to say 'no' when needed. Make time for relaxation, perhaps meditation, and some exercise during the week. This is important when preparing for pregnancy because stress can negatively impact on female hormones and even switch off ovulation.

9. Take a good multivitamin and mineral supplement aimed at improving egg quality and hormone balance. It should contain folic acid, a good amount of zinc and B vitamins.

10. Don't delay . . . even if your menstrual cycle is regular it is not a guarantee that you are ovulating or that the quality of your eggs is optimal.

# CHAPTER 6

## *Restorative Yoga and Mindful Movement*

It is common for the body to grow tense when experiencing fertility-related physical examinations or giving oneself injections of hormones, and this can increase feelings of disconnect from our physical self. Discomfort and pain, or thoughts that our body isn't doing what it 'should' do, exacerbate feelings of mistrusting our body. The mind continues to be busy and plan while the body feels tired and ill at ease. When our mind is out of rhythm with our body, we have the potential to experience 'burnout'; a form of physical and mental exhaustion that is not so easy to recover from. When our mind and body are not in sync it can also influence how we connect to our partner and treatment approaches, such as TSI, become mechanical rather than intimate and pleasurable experiences (see page 77). Reconnecting with your body through movement and mindfulness is healing on a physical and emotional level and supports you to work through fertility-related issues in a more embodied way, with mind, body and spirit working in harmony.

Restorative yoga is a form of physical movement that focuses on the healing potential of exercise, rather than overusing our muscles and aiming to push them to their limits. It works with what feels natural for our body and reduces the physiological response we experience when we are stressed. The physicality of exercising in this way includes a focus on body alignment and has been attributed to improving muscle and joint health, as well as benefiting the cardiovascular system and normalizing blood-sugar levels, promoting hormone balance. This form of exercise also supports a reduction in inflammation and an improved immune system, naturally beneficial to fertility health.

Restorative yoga allows the body to move its muscles in a variety of poses while practising breathing techniques to support you in holding the movements mindfully and for extended periods of time. In theory, you are exercising the body while stilling the mind.

As you reconnect to your body, you release mind and body tension and tend to move towards increased self-care with more self-compassion. With this approach, it is often easier to face any fertility-related difficulties in day-to-day living.

## Restorative Yoga Poses or Asanas

The yoga pose sequences in restorative yoga include forward folds, gentle twists, chest or 'heart' openers, and pelvic-floor exercises to help tone muscle and release tension. The Asanas are supported with the use of two yoga blocks, one or two yoga bolsters and a blanket/pillow to ease you into the postures and promote relaxation. This basic yoga equipment can be sourced easily from a yoga centre, sports shop or online.

Asanas are combined with breathwork techniques (known as Pranayama) to support the sympathetic nervous system and create an internal emotional balance. This is beneficial as there are many fluctuating emotions associated with fertility problems, including sadness, joy, frustration, relief, distress, envy, worry, anxiety, enthusiasm, surprise, guilt and despair, to name a few!

Restorative yoga creates a release from tension within your body and mind. It aims to promote deep relaxation within and enables you to let go of mental stress.

\* **Please note:** as with any exercise, there can be contraindications for particular conditions or illnesses, for example, those with degenerative bone disease, retinal, heart or spine/neck problems. It is also recommended not to practice postures which are contraindicated in the first trimester of pregnancy or that bring pressure to your pelvic area. It is recommended that you seek the advice of your medical practitioner as to the suitability of undertaking any exercise programme or restorative yoga if you have any medical condition that contraindicates such exercise.

### Top Tips for Restorative Yoga

1. **Prepare your props.** Ensure that you have the necessary props ready: two yoga blocks, a yoga mat, one or two yoga bolsters, one blanket, one yoga strap and two sandbags.
2. **Be your own caregiver;** adopting an attitude of being your own caregiver will deepen a sense of self-compassion as you guide yourself through the poses.
3. **Hold your space** by practising at the same time each day – the beginning or end of your day will promote rejuvenation and rest. You could alternate between sitting meditation and restorative yoga if you are time limited.

4. **Let your props support you;** restorative yoga is a healing process. The props help to stabilize and support each pose and reduce the effort involved in maintaining them, for example, the strap does the work of holding your leg in position rather than you overstretching and losing the position. The bolster and sandbags help to hold you in the pose.

5. **Create a mindful space.** Ideally, practise your yoga poses in a light and clear space. Using a 'less-is-more' approach will offer more opportunity for clarity of mind rather than finding a small space in a crowded room, which would tend to feel more chaotic. You can also use a mindful bell or chime (often available to download as an app for a computer or smartphone) to indicate when the pose is coming to a close so that you can move harmoniously from one pose into the next.

6. **Don't overexert yourself.** It is often instinctual to aim to stretch more and push your body to go further. Our culture encourages us from a young age to be competitive and to do and achieve more. In contrast, in restorative yoga once you achieve a pose you are encouraged to stay with it rather than try to do more. It can feel uncomfortable to let go physically if you are used to being a 'must do' busy person. The intention is to develop a deep sense of ease, gained by connecting to a more neutral sensation – one of self-care – rather than striving for better.

The following restorative yoga sequence is aimed at grounding and soothing your body. It can bring some welcome healing, especially when going through the rigours of fertility testing and treatment. An anxious body can lead to an anxious or depressed mind and paying attention to reducing the tension in our body leads to the mind feeling calm and alert. The breathwork used helps to elicit the relaxation response, which in turn calms our nervous system. You will also begin to connect deeper into your physical rather than thinking self with each breath.

You may wish to complete the whole sequence or do one or two of the poses in the sequence at a time. Allow your body to let you know what it needs and how much is too much.

## The Healing Breath Exercise

This breath exercise is straightforward and will help in easing internal tension as it calms the nervous system. You can also use it before your restorative yoga practice to slow the mind and body.

Practising this exercise helps the body to self-soothe, reducing feelings of panic or fear. This breathwork can be used when attending scans or other medical procedures which may need to be undertaken as part of your fertility treatment.

- Sit comfortably with your back in an upright position.
- Position your tongue towards the roof of your mouth and place the tip at the back of your front teeth.
- Drop your jaw, while still holding your tongue in place, at the back of your teeth. Breathe out fully through your mouth.
- Now close your mouth with your tongue still in place and inhale deeply through your nose.
- Once you have inhaled, hold your breath for 3, 2, 1.
- Exhale slowly and release, holding your mouth open and your tongue positioned as before at the tip of the tissue behind your front teeth.
- Repeat this deep breath inhale and exhale three times.

### Diaphragmatic Breathwork in Relaxation Pose

You can move easily from the healing breath exercise into more yoga-focused diaphragmatic breathing. Awareness-focused breath-work is an important component of restorative yoga as it eases you into the pose. Taking natural, long and deep breaths into the abdominal area and letting go of those breaths as though releasing them from the entire body helps to bring your body back into balance.

- On the exhale, breathe out for slightly longer to support a further reduction in internal stress.
- When breathing in slowly, notice the intake of breath at the tips of your nostrils and how it moves through your body.
- Rest your hands on your abdomen and feel the movement of the breath as your stomach inflates and deflates with each breath.
- Stay in this pose for longer if you want to benefit from deeper relaxation.

Combine diaphragmatic breathing with the following relaxation pose:

Duration:      10 minutes (set your mindful bell reminder)
Yoga props:   yoga mat
                      bolster
                      3 blankets
                      eye pillow or hand towel folded three times

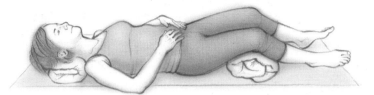

Relaxation Pose with Diaphragmatic Breathing

- Position a blanket (folded three times) on the mat to support your head.
- Before you lie flat on your back on your yoga mat, place the bolster underneath the back of your knees so they rest on it. You may also require another folded blanket, positioned lengthways from the top of your head to the end of the lumbar region of your spine, to provide further support to your lower spine. If you find that your neck is hyper-extended and feeling uncomfortable, you could place a further blanket folded three times under your head with the folded end at your shoulder area and allow your shoulders to drop down into the mat.
- You may wish to keep your hands on your tummy area to notice the in- and out-breaths, or at a slight angle (approximately 35 degrees) from your side, resting with your palms facing up.
- You can place an eye pillow or folded hand towel over your eyes for light blackout if you feel comfortable doing so. This can promote deeper rest. However, for some this may

feel too exposing and could increase feelings of vulnerability. Weighting is also used in restorative exercise to help you feel more grounded; you can add an extra bolster or place two blankets folded three times across your abdomen in addition to your eye pillow.

◆ Begin your diaphragmatic breathing as you lie flat, facing upwards, and settle deeper into your reclined lying position. Notice where any areas of tension are in your body and direct your breath towards these areas. Notice also how your body and, in particular, your spine, connects with the mat underneath. You may notice that your mind is active with thoughts or beginning to experience some inner tranquillity. Just observe your sensations, feelings and thoughts without becoming overly engaged with them. Allow yourself to let go of mental activity. Notice thoughts as though they are clouds passing in the sky.

◆ After holding this pose for 10 minutes, you may wish to extend it to move into a supported bridge pose.

## Supported Bridge Pose

Extending into a supported bridge pose helps to release any tension in the hip flexors. It also expands the muscles in the chest and abdominal area, a part of our body often associated with stress retention, especially when administering hormone injections for IVF.

Duration:     5–10 minutes (set your mindful bell reminder)
Yoga props:   yoga mat
              bolster
              1 blanket
              yoga belt (or any cloth strap that can be tied)

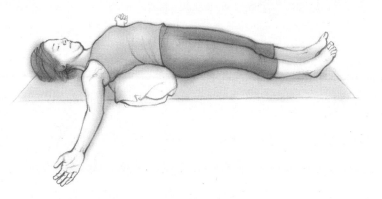

Supported Bridge Pose

- Place the bolster sideways on the yoga mat to provide support to your lower back and hip area while your buttocks and hips are lifted gently off the ground, as outlined below.

- Place a rolled blanket, sideways, directly beside the bolster which will further support your lower back. Ensure that the whole lower back and hip area are supported as your spine and hips are lifted off the mat on the in-breath and rested down on the support on the out-breath.

- Keep your legs a hip distance apart with your ankles resting flat on the mat. Recline into the supported bridge pose by curling your spine off the mat and on to your support bolster and blanket one vertebra at a time.

- Breathe naturally and place your arms out to the side with the palms facing upwards towards the roof. Your shoulders should rest into the mat. Ensure that your head and neck are also supported with the mat beneath. Having the chest area raised slightly higher than your head deepens relaxation.

- After 10 minutes, turn your head sideways and roll slowly on to your side, sweeping your arm across your chest to place your hand flat on the side of the mat for extra support when sitting up.

- To loosen up your back and hip area, move into a supine twist pose.

## Supine Twist Pose

Duration:      5 minutes (set your mindful bell reminder)
Yoga props:  yoga mat (move your other props slightly out
              of reach)

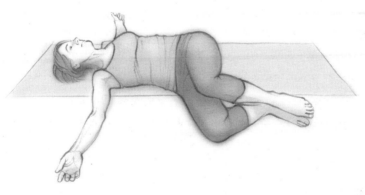

Supine Twist Pose

* Lie flat on your back on your yoga mat.
* Place your arms stretched out at shoulder height with your
  hands facing upwards.
* As you inhale, bring your legs together, bending your
  knees. Raise them up with your feet flat on the ground.
* As you exhale move your legs (still bent) to the right, resting them on the other side of the mat (if possible, without

overstretching). Keep your head turned to the left. On the inhale, return your knees to centre with your feet on the ground and also moving your head to neutral position, with your eyes looking towards the ceiling. Now, repeat the exercise, moving your legs (bent) to the left and your head slowly turning to the right. Repeat these movements for 5 minutes breathing naturally. If you get lost in thought or sensations, take your attention back to mindfully being present to the rotation from right to neutral, and then to the left and back.

- When you have finished the exercise, stretch out on the mat: stretch your arms and hands above your head and feel the full-body stretch as you straighten your legs down, resting on the mat on the exhale. Before moving on to the next pose, you can stay in the lying position and move into some deeper muscle relaxation with the progressive muscle relaxation exercise below.

## Progressive Muscle Relaxation Exercise

Progressive muscle relaxation (PMR) was developed by an American physician and psychiatrist, Dr Edmund Jacobson, in the 1920s.[1] This exercise aims to engage tension in the muscles and then relax them at a deeper level, contrasting tension with relaxation in each muscle group progressively. Daily life stresses are often carried in our body and we do not necessarily notice the levels of tension increasing. Whether you are aiming to be at a 9am clinic appointment and wondering what time you will reach your office or you are about to take your long-awaited pregnancy test, PMR helps you to recognize how you are responding physically and release any muscular tension that you are holding.

Duration:    15–20 minutes (set your mindful bell reminder)
Yoga props:  yoga mat

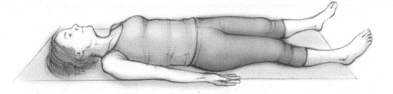

Progressive Muscle Relaxation

- Lying flat on your yoga mat, stretch out as best you can, and place your arms parallel to your body with the hands facing up towards the ceiling. This exercise will involve focusing on each muscle group.
- Begin by taking a deep breath in and imagining the breath being drawn all the way down your body. As you exhale, have an intention to 'let go' of all the tension being carried.
- Take 3 deep inhales and exhales in this way.
- Now begin your muscle tensing by clenching your fists, holding them in a tight fist and counting back slowly 5-4-3-2-1 in your mind. Then release the hold and spread your fingers out, counting 1-2-3-4-5 slowly as you do so.
- Now bring your awareness to your biceps and forearms and tense the muscles as tightly as you can, again holding this tension for 5–1 and slowly release as fully as you can, holding again for 1–5. Remember to breathe as deeply as you can.
- Now bring your attention to your shoulders and draw your shoulder blades towards each other, holding them tense for 5–1 and relaxing them down and releasing fully for 1–5. Now become aware of the muscles either side of your spine and around your lower back. When you are muscle tensing this area, your lower back will naturally curve. Allow this to happen and hold the tension in your whole back area for 5–1 and release for 1–5.
- Moving down the body, focus your attention on your buttocks area, squeezing your muscles and holding together for 5–1 and then releasing fully for 1–5.
- Now, become aware of your pelvis area and tense around here and the hips, really feeling the tension in your protective hip/pelvis area. Hold this, squeezing for 5–1 and release for 1–5.

- Gently move on to the top of your legs and particularly tense the back of your thighs. Then tense the muscles at the front of your thighs, down to your knees, holding then releasing. It can help to focus the tension from the knees up to the top of your leg rather than from the top down.

- Moving down the leg, squeeze the muscles at the back of your legs and around the front of the shin bone area. If sitting, this can be helped by raising your legs out in front of you and focusing on tensing the lower leg area. You raise your feet and legs slightly off the ground. By pulling the toes back towards you, the muscles in your calves will naturally tighten. Once again, hold this area tense for 5–1 and release for 1–5.

- Now moving on to your feet, curl your toes back towards your feet and feel the muscle tension in your feet. Hold the tension in your foot for 5–1 and release for 1–5.

- Now take your attention back to the front of your body, around your abdomen area. Tighten your stomach and pull the muscles gently towards your back, holding for 5–1, and gently releasing for 1–5.

- Move up along your body around your ribs, feeling the intercostal muscle group, and as you breathe in, hold the muscles tense, feeling your ribcage rise with the in-breath and release on the out-breath. As you focus on the ribs rising and falling with the in- and out-breaths, gently take your attention to the chest area.

- Hold the chest muscles tense for 5–1 and then relax fully into the mat for 1–5. Hold and release.

- Taking your attention to your shoulder area, tighten all the muscles and then draw your shoulders towards your ears, holding for 5–1 and then releasing, dropping your shoulders and being with that sensation for 1–5.

- Moving upwards focus your attention on to your neck and tense the entire neck area for 5–1. Then release for 1–5. If you have any physical problems with your neck area, avoid this and move directly on to your jaw area. If not, draw your head up and back, resting the top area of your head on the mat. You can extend the area by raising your chin so your neck is stretched fully and, once again, tense and release the entire neck area.

- Now take your attention to the muscles around your jaw. Open your mouth fully, tensing and stretching the connecting muscles in front of your ears on both sides of your head. Hold them tense for 5–1 and then release the hold fully for 1–5.

- Moving away from the jaw area, tighten the muscles around your eyes by squeezing them tightly shut for 5–1 and releasing the tension for 1–5.

- Also, tighten your cheeks and forehead. Raise your eyebrows, hold for 2 seconds and release. Repeat this 3 times.

- Now imagine tensing your entire head area and feel the weight of the tension being held, hold for 5–1 and then relax fully for 1–5.

- You can end the PMR exercise by taking 3 deep breaths in and releasing fully on the out-breath, while holding a sense of your body as a whole.

You can then move your body closer to the wall to move into the gentle inversion pose.

## Gentle Inversion Pose

Inversion poses help to increase balance and relieve stress. They are also recommended to aid circulation and increase concentration. As with most yoga poses, they are beneficial to both mind and body. It is worth noting that inversion poses are generally not recommended to undertake during menstruation.

Duration: 10 minutes (set your mindful bell reminder)
Yoga props: yoga mat
1 blanket
eye pillow (optional)
yoga sandbag or bolster

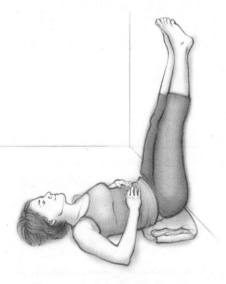

Gentle Inversion Pose

- Place your mat with its width directly against the wall. Place your yoga props within easy reach.
- Sit on your mat sideways, positioning your left hip close to the wall while keeping your legs bent. Support your back by turning in a sweeping motion, moving your legs up the length of the wall while you are leaning back to lie flat on the length of your mat. This gets easier to do with practice!
- As your torso is flat against the mat, position your buttocks as close to the wall as you can without discomfort, while your legs are positioned straight up against the wall.
- If you feel an overstretch in your hamstrings, move your buttocks slightly away from the wall.
- This slight inversion pose can be further elevated by placing a blanket folded 4 times directly under the buttocks to slightly raise the abdomen area causing it to lean slightly towards your heart.
- Finally, place a sandbag (or yoga bolster) on the soles of your flat feet, facing the roof. This optional weighting helps you to feel more grounded while also releasing the hips and lower back.
- To deepen the experience, you can reduce sensory stimulation by covering your eyes with an eye pillow or hand towel folded 3 times.
- Remain in this position for up to 10 minutes before easing yourself away from the wall by bending your legs and gently pushing upwards on the mat and away from the wall. Move to the side with the support of one arm flat on the ground and one arm bent across the body, hand flat on the mat as you push yourself up sideways to sitting position.
- You can then gently roll yourself into the nurturing child's pose.

## Child's Pose

The child's pose helps you to feel supported and grounded; it is very calming. Maintain physical comfort throughout and allow yourself time in the pose to deepen the benefit.

Duration:     5–10 minutes (set your mindful bell reminder)

Yoga props:  yoga mat

                bolster, or pillow rolled in half

                1 or 2 blankets

                towel folded 3 times

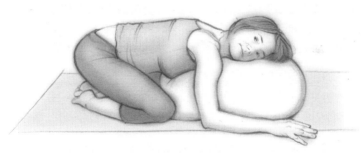

Child's Pose

* Begin by placing the bolster in the centre of the mat lengthways and positioning yourself behind it, facing towards it.

- Kneel with your knees a little more than hip width apart and sit on your heels.
- Do a quick body scan and notice any areas of discomfort in your knees, legs or hips. Adjust your position to bring additional comfort to these areas.
- With your knees and legs held in their position, lean forward gently to rest on the bolster. Your head is positioned turned to the left or right, towards the top of the bolster. Your forearms are resting on the mat with your elbows directly beneath the shoulders.
- Your hips and your head are level with the bolster creating support under your torso. If your head is significantly lower than your hips, you may wish to fold a blanket in quarters and place it lengthways on the bolster to increase height. If you are very tall, you could add an extra bolster.
- You may wish to support your feet by placing a towel folded 3 times under your ankles. For additional support, you can also place a soft blanket under your knees.
- If you experience tightness in your hips, add a small pillow behind your knees, raising your upper legs slightly and providing more support.
- Rest your head to the side. If this is uncomfortable, you may wish to cross your forearms and place your forehead directly on them, facing down.
- During this pose you take deep breaths in and exhale fully and for longer to help deepen the relaxation.
- Use a mindfulness timed bell, or some other non-intrusive alarm, to indicate that you have completed the 5–10-minute child's pose. This is a gentle and nurturing pose to bring this restorative yoga sequence to a close.

## Mindful Walking Meditation

You can also bring conscious awareness to your movement away from your yoga space with some mindful walking meditation. This can also replace some of your restorative yoga sequence if you are limited for time and in another location. We are often rushing from one place to the next, or one job to another, and get lost in the mental activity associated with planning. Mindful walking is a reflective alternative to sitting meditation and can be used at different times throughout your day: while waiting for your train or when taking time out in the park or countryside.

As with restorative yoga exercise, mindful movement aims to contribute towards an inner ease, rather than journeying from A to B with determination and a spring in your step, which of course is also necessary at times! Always being in a hurry can add extra internal stress to a challenging experience. Whether you are walking from a consultant's office to a waiting room or from your desk to the conference room, mindful walking allows you to connect and focus on your body muscles, feelings and sensations while you are in motion. Doing this even once a day in a nine-to-five job ensures that you have taken some moments to check-in with yourself, something that is often forgotten when you are meeting other needs. Mindful movement helps to focus the mind and provide clarity of thought, supporting you to respond rather than react to the immediate stimulus.

Although it may seem relatively easy to slow down your body rhythm, it can be challenging. If you are feeling agitated or distracted, the tendency is to want to move faster rather than to slow down and relax into your body.

- As you move from sitting to standing position, do so with slow intention, noticing each part of your body rising to support you. Focus on your ankles, calf and upper leg muscles as you lift your body to standing position.
- Drop your shoulders down and notice your shoulder blades relax into position. Really sense all the movement involved in your body standing.
- Begin walking slowly with a clear and present focus to each movement. Notice how the soles of your feet connect to the ground beneath and how you shift all your weight on to your left foot, leg, hip, and how you move into placing your weight on to your right foot, leg, hip. Become involved in the daily experience of walking which we often miss and take for granted.
- As your body connects with the earth beneath, begin to stay present to the 'now' moment of walking.
- Although you may have a strong urge to move faster, notice the urge and rather than automatically following it, deliberately slow the pace of your movement, balancing the weight down into both feet. Feel your feet as they connect to your shoes and notice how they are supported by the earth beneath. Help to feel grounded in the connection of your feet slowly moving you forward.
- Notice any mental chatter or judgement urging you to move on or to abandon this experience.
- Congratulate yourself for allowing yourself some time to be present to what is happening within.
- Slowly move your feet and feel each step connect.
- Consciously lift each leg, feel it move forward and reconnect once again with the ground beneath. Notice each

small movement involved in walking as you move your weight from left to right in the motion of walking.

- You may begin to notice that you are carrying feelings or sensations in areas of your body. These feelings may be associated with inner judgement or feared judgement from others. You may also notice that you are carrying positive feelings such as calm, joy or excitement. Just observe these feelings as being present and take your attention back to the slow and conscious awareness of walking.

- Breathe in to each movement, taking slow deep breaths in through the nose and exhaling out through the mouth. If you are carrying tension in your jaw muscles, gently drop the hold and allow your mouth to drop open slightly.

- Notice when your mind wanders, calling your attention with demands or fantasy thoughts. Just notice these thoughts and return your focus back to the slow and deliberate felt experience of mindful walking.

- If your mind is very busy, you may wish to repeat an internal cue such as 'walking slowly, walking slowly' as you match your breath to the slow and intentioned movement.

- When you reach your intended destination (although with mindful movement, you don't always need a destination, for example, it may be mindful walking in your garden or in a park), take 3 deep breaths. Breathe as though taking the breath from the top of your body all the way down to your feet on the inhale, and from the soles of your feet to the top of your head on the exhale. Notice any added stillness or calm within. Take this with you to your next activity and allow clarity of mind to follow.

- Try this every day for 5–10 minutes.

You can vary this mindful walking meditation by focusing on the environment, rather than your internal process, while you walk. Really connect with the colours, textures and shapes in your immediate environment. If you are passing trees, notice the deep colour of the leaves or the rugged texture of the tree branches above. If you are passing buildings, notice the shop windows and the shapes and colours of all you pass as you take in your environment with the eyes of a painter new to their landscape.

As you walk slowly, also pay close attention to the texture of the ground beneath, the smells (pleasant and unpleasant) and the sounds that move closer and further into the distance. Become present to the sensations of warm or cool air against your face and skin as you move with integrated ease within your environment.

### Journal Activity: Self-care

- How comfortable am I about looking after my own needs?
- How do I feel when I take care of my needs?
- When giving time to self-care, what thoughts do I notice, for example, 'I should be doing something else', etc.
- Do I believe that self-care and non-striving are also helpful to my emotional well-being? If yes, expand . . . If no, where did I learn this belief? Is my belief helpful? What are the gains and losses of holding on to this belief?

- How did I feel before my restorative yoga; emotionally and psychologically? If there were strong feelings, name the feeling (for example, anxious, sad, excited). Where did I feel these feelings in my body and how present were they on a scale of 0–10 (0 = not present, 10 = strongly present).
- How did I feel after my restorative yoga or mindful movement; emotionally and psychologically? Did I notice any change to my feelings? How do they feel now on a scale of 0–10?

You may wish to build on your restorative yoga practice by joining a class and benefitting from working within a group environment. If you can't locate a restorative yoga class near to you, Hatha yoga would also be beneficial. Avoid joining any high-impact classes (for example, hot yoga). The aim of yoga in a fertility support context is to help your body feel rejuvenated and relaxed. Like the next chapter on understanding and changing your thinking with CBT, you can decide whether you need to deepen your experience further with group or individual support.

CHAPTER 7

# Fertility Thinking with Cognitive Behavioural Therapy

Managing fertility problems can challenge even the most optimistic of minds. A natural desire to have a child begins with pleasant imaginings of decorating the nursery and choosing baby names, and leads to feelings of hope and excitement. When faced with fertility difficulties, however, dreams of a hoped-for child can fade into increased feelings of anxiety and pressure with each passing month. Of course, for many the dream of a family will be realized, while sadly others may try without success. It is the uncertainty of how long it will take, what they will physically, psychologically and financially need to endure and if or when they may need treatment that causes increased levels of distress for these couples and individuals.

Most major life changes carry an element of stress, even when they are pleasant: how many people have you seen stressed in airports on the first day of their holiday? Investing in the physical aspects of treating fertility problems can be all-consuming and, as a result, your emotional and psychological needs can easily get pushed down your list of priorities. However, taking care of your mind health both benefits your body and provides you with the much-needed resilience and self-kindness that will see you through your fertility journey.

Calming the mind can begin at any point before, during or after you embark on natural or assisted fertility treatment. It helps to provide clarity of mind in the decision-making process and also reconnects you to your 'real' or authentic self, meaning you are more centred and less swayed by the ups and downs of trying for a baby. Looking after your mind health also has the added benefit of calming the internal struggle that can so often accompany the process.

Often when feeling stressed or low, we get caught in over-thinking or become overwhelmed by emotions. While it is important to allow ourselves to feel, it is unhelpful if we are unable to release ourselves from challenging feelings, for example, shame, guilt, depression or fear, as they can stop us from progressing towards our goals. It is hard to look to the future or accept past events if we combine them with a harsh inner dialogue full of self-blame. It is easy to see how such thinking can lead to increased feelings of stress, sleep disturbance, irritability or an inability to be with our situation, for example, constantly rushing around seeking reassurance from others, which may also include seeking many medical opinions rather than making a decision after a reasonable amount of medical assessment. It can also lead to strained relationships with family, colleagues and friends.

Managing infertility problems can be one of the most challenging times for an individual or couple. Before booking the first appointment with a consultant for fertility support, most have already experienced worries accompanied by a range of thoughts that can be filled with self-doubt and fear for the future. This can mean that even before any solution is sought, the individual feels overcome by powerful negative feelings, which can include low mood, grief, anxiety, unhealthy envy, loss of self-esteem, or fear and guilt towards their partner or close family members, for example, 'Why can't I give my parents the grandchild they so want?'

There are several straightforward cognitive behavioural techniques that will enable you to change self-sabotaging beliefs, reduce stress and ultimately support you in making choices that help improve treatment outcomes, and these are outlined in detail below.

## Minding your Mind with Cognitive Behavioural Therapy

The connection between how we think and how we feel is well established in the field of psychological health, and positive change is commonly supported using a form of therapy known as cognitive behavioural therapy (CBT). Cognitive behavioural therapy focuses on our thinking, how this contributes to the way we feel and our corresponding behaviour, for example, what we do or what we avoid doing because we think and feel the way we do. It is a form of therapy that encourages us to not just express our thoughts and feelings, but to be more objective with our thinking to help us to actively change what we're doing and how we're feeling. Cognitive behavioural therapy supports the individual to establish more self-supportive ways of thinking, which in turn contribute to improved feelings and a more positive approach to the situations and relationships in our daily life. Cognitive behavioural therapy is research-based and has been listed in the UK's guidelines for best practice in healthcare as an effective therapy, approved in the treatment of a range of psychological issues, including stress, anxiety, low mood, depression and thinking styles that can lead to unhealthy anger or envy.

I often describe CBT as a therapy that trains you to be your own therapist as it requires that you actively monitor your thoughts and feelings in certain trigger situations, for example, when asked by a family member if you're ever going to start a family, long after you have been attending treatment! It supports you in establishing change when you recognize unhelpful thinking styles and, as it is a solution-focused therapy, it draws on your innate ability to bring balance to your thoughts and feelings to help you make wise decisions.

It is important to understand that being solution-focused does not mean that we create unrealistic expectations. For example, if I visualize winning the lottery, it may not mean that I win it next week, however, I will begin to create the life that I would like if I had won it: travel more, enjoy living more and take appropriate self-care in negative situations or relationships. When we are only focused on the negative, we do not notice the other areas of our life that support us or that are working well. Our mind has incredible power over how we feel and what we do to a positive and negative effect.

### Exposing the Myths about Cognitive Behavioural Therapy

- **CBT will work instantly and changes lifelong habits in weeks**
  CBT is like any new change – it requires ongoing effort to create lasting change. Cognitive behavioural therapy will provide you with the skills and support to understand and change thinking habits and, like increasing your fitness in the gym, you will need to flex your mind muscles for lasting change!

- **CBT doesn't allow you to feel**
  Using CBT will not mean that you don't feel. It simply helps you not to be overwhelmed by an emotional response, which can mean that you are making decisions or avoiding situations just to avoid the feelings associated with them. This is helpful if this is in your best interest but perhaps unhelpful if your emotions begin to drive your decision-making processes, for example, you may decide to avoid going to seek fertility-related tests because you feel anxious about the result. Naturally, this decreases the anxiety in the short term but contributes to a longer-term anxiety that can be more difficult to be with.

> ### ● CBT does not explore the past
>
> Cognitive behavioural therapy will explore experiences in the past and will gain from this understanding to focus on how it influences the present. In other words, because that happened, how does it make you feel now, or what do you do in relationships now because of a past relationship, etc.? This way the focus is on how to positively change, using your resources in the present, to experience a more rewarding difference moving forward.

Often, our way of responding to events in our present is informed by our past, and it is important to understand why we may feel 'shame' or 'guilt' relating to our fertility. For example, if you grew up in a family where you were not given the space for emotional expression or where there were excessive emotional responses to events (for example, immense anger or emotional breakdowns), you might respond in a similar way when faced with a challenging time. Cognitive behavioural therapy for fertility is not focused on keeping you in a place where you would continuously reflect on this over many months; instead it invites you to recognize where this type of feeling (for example, shame) relates to your experience in the present, where it also may have been influenced from the past and, most importantly, how to release and change this in response to things now. Past events are drawn on only to inform a healthy and self-supportive approach to present challenging circumstances. A catharsis of feeling can be the basis by which we learn that we are suffering and may need some support. Cognitive behavioural therapy can help us to respond rather than react to triggering events that remind us in some way of a previous difficulty in our life. An example could be not feeling any joy with a positive pregnancy result because of experiencing a previous pregnancy loss. This is completely understandable and needs to be worked through. However, it can also be helped by understanding and changing some of our thinking patterns so that we can experience more hope and joy with our positive breakthroughs.

While it provides the space to be present to your experience, CBT also suggests areas where you can integrate positive changes and try them out in similar situations, for example, if you feel anxious every time you meet with your acupuncturist or consultant, CBT would explore what internal dialogue and beliefs are present during these events and if any of them hinder your goal of helpful communication. It would show you how you might change your thoughts to be more self-empowering. You would then practise the new thinking style in future appointments. This very active approach is why CBT is often referred to as a 'directive' therapy. By identifying unhelpful thinking patterns, CBT can enable you to replace them with more self-supportive thinking styles by working with 'thought records' (see page 178) and 'positive self-statements' (see page 181), combined with changing what you do during times of challenge.

Cognitive behavioural therapy also helps you to recognize when you have established deep-held beliefs leading to wounds that you then carry forward, for example, instead of seeing the IVF cycle as having failed, you begin to believe 'I am a failure', which can then be carried forward along with its associated limiting thoughts and feelings of loss and putting yourself down (known as 'self-downing').

## Changing Unhelpful Thinking Patterns

Our thinking styles can become ingrained and quickly turn into the lens through which we habitually experience our situations. Watch out for the following patterns of thinking, ones which CBT pioneer, Albert Ellis, identified as being the root cause of excessive feelings of distress:

- **Catastrophizing:** the language we use when we are in this thinking style contributes to stress and anxiety; 'I can't cope', 'It's always going to be like this.' It usually jumps quickly to the worst-case scenario: 'IVF only ever works for other people; it will never work for us.'

- **Fortune telling:** in fortune telling, we assume that we know our future and it usually ends badly! 'If this does not happen for me, my partner will leave me.' Often fortune telling is present even if there is only minimal evidence and a person couples this with other disappointments in their past to validate their belief that the future is bleak.

- **Mind reading:** like fortune telling, mind reading is not an ability that we generally possess! However, in times of stress we can believe that we will know how everyone will respond. An example could be the need to take time off work for a visit to a clinic; 'My boss is clearly judging me and won't have any understanding if I let him know I need to attend a consultation.' While this may be true, mind reading usually doesn't offer an alternative perspective. It is important not to believe your mind-reading abilities 100 per cent and to engage with assertive communication skills instead.

- **Over focusing on the negative and not acknowledging the positive:** 'Nothing good happens to us,' etc. It is important to write about all the areas of your life – friendships, career, relationship with partner, health and hobbies/interests, spiritual self – and acknowledge what is working, to resource yourself for the area that is currently very challenging (for example, fertility health). Only in doing so do we feel resourced to manage these difficulties as they present themselves.

- **Believing your 'shoulds':** the tyranny of 'shoulds' can be constant, particularly if you discover that you need treatment you weren't expecting. 'This should not be happening,' 'I should have known this sooner and acted on planning a family ten years ago.' 'Shoulds' are usually demands we make of ourselves without first exploring why we may have chosen a route, for example, 'I did not know I had a fertility-related problem until now and I can only make a choice to treat something I know I have.'

- **Blaming:** the fertility road can be bumpy at times, causing us inner turmoil as we try to work out the next step and get over some real disappointments. As we try to make sense of what is happening, we can begin to internalize or externalize the hurt. This can be very subtle but can cause us to feel even more depressed – 'It's my fault; if I hadn't worked through my last cycle it would have worked, I was too busy, I'm to blame for all of this.' The frustration can also be projected on to our partner – 'Why isn't he feeling the way I do?' or 'It's her fault anyway and now she can't cope with it, why should I deal with this?' It is important to let go of this way of thinking as it can quickly erode self-confidence and damage your relationship.

*

By changing how you talk to yourself in stressful situations (internally), you can heal much quicker and regain a sense of equilibrium. Instead of depression you would experience sadness after a negative event, which is more manageable. Instead of anxiety you may experience concern, which helps you rather than hinders you in your fertility process. Instead of feeling out of control as unhealthy anger can sometimes make you feel ('It's his/her/the clinic's fault and I will let everybody know'), a different perspective may lead to healthier anger ('I don't like this and there needs to be change'), leading to making better choices moving forward and expressing your needs appropriately, without the feelings lingering.

### Release Negative Thoughts

Over the next week, begin to notice if you tend to fall into any of the thinking patterns outlined above, relating to your fertility experiences. For example, just notice if you are catastrophizing or fortune telling. If there is a trend in your thinking, you can begin releasing yourself from negative habitual thinking styles by working with CBT thought records and challenging unhelpful thoughts.

While it is completely natural to have negative thoughts and feelings, particularly when experiencing a crisis, left unchallenged they can deepen the burden of the experience. It is important to manage fertility-related problems and associated tests and treatment with as much self-compassion and equilibrium as possible. It is helpful to recognize and find a new internal dialogue when you may be being judgemental towards yourself, your partner or what you need to face. It also helps to gain a balanced perspective which contributes positively to decision-making processes, for example, whether a particular treatment approach is for you or not. It is useful to track unhelpful, automatic (because they pop in when you're not expecting them!) thoughts and start to challenge them. Begin to become more aware of the fertility-related thoughts you are experiencing and track them in your thought record (see page 178). These thoughts may be positive ('We are taking a supportive step towards helping our fertility problem'), negative ('This is hopeless') or neutral ('I'll wear this top with my jeans today to the clinic'). By becoming aware of your internal dialogue in trigger situations, you can begin to challenge and change the unhelpful thinking patterns and find a more self-supportive internal dialogue. This has also been shown to change how we feel. The thoughts listed below include elements of self-downing, putting down others (known as 'other-downing'), over-generalizing, over-personalizing and catastrophizing. It is easy to perceive how, left unchallenged, feelings of frustration, anger, depression or anxiety could increase.

Negative automatic fertility-related thoughts could include any of the following in times of stress:

- 'People absolutely should be sensitive to our situation and stop asking me when we're planning to have children.' *(Other-downing, even when they don't know that you're experiencing difficulty!)*
- 'Everyone else has an easier life.' *(Over-generalizing)*
- 'My partner should leave me as he'd have a better life without me.' *(Self-downing and fortune telling)*

- 'This cycle has to be successful or I'm a failure.' (*Self-downing*)
- 'Other women drink and smoke and still give birth. Life shouldn't be like this.' (*All-or-nothing thinking – things are absolute with no grey areas*)
- 'I left it too late.' (*Over-personalizing – holding yourself responsible for things when you didn't have information; you didn't know there was a medical problem earlier*)
- 'This is my/his/her fault.' (*Self-/other-downing – fertility problems are a physical medical problem and not a choice*)
- 'I can't cope without a baby. Life will not be worth living.' (*Catastrophizing and discounting the positives – this is a particularly challenging way of thinking as it can lead to feelings of deep depression*)

## Your Thought Record

Begin to track your thoughts in the thought record below. If you are not quite sure what you are thinking in situations, you can begin by placing yellow stickies around your home in significant places, for example, on the bathroom mirror, on the fridge, on the TV, on your car dashboard, etc. When you see them it can prompt you to recognize your internal dialogue: 'What am I saying to myself right now?' Notice when you have strayed into all-or-nothing thinking, for example, 'Oh no, I can't cope with being late for work, this is a disaster', in response to hearing about a train strike on the news!

# Fertility-Related Thought Record

| Trigger situation relating to my fertility | Unhelpful thoughts or beliefs that were prompted ... And what I wanted to do when I felt this way ... | Describe the feelings you had because of this | Self-compassionate alternatives to thoughts or beliefs that were triggered | What can I do differently in this situation, if not now, in the future? | How do I feel now? Take a breath and notice where you connect to this feeling in your body. |
|---|---|---|---|---|---|
| Where were you; with whom? | When this happened, what were you thinking? | Name the feeling and rate how strongly you feel it on a scale of 0-10 (10 being the strongest). | Is there another way to look at this? | Is there anything that I do which is not helpful to me in that situation? | Becoming aware of our feelings and where we experience them in our bodies allows us to be more present. It can help to create a pause between our stressors and how we respond to our stressors. Stop, breathe, notice and respond (not react). |
| What happened in detail? | What do you believe about yourself or others, for example, your partner, because this happened? | Where do you notice it in your body? | What would you say to a good friend if they were in this situation? | What could I do differently now or in the future? | Note where you carry uncomfortable feelings in your body: your head, your stomach or chest area? |
| When did this occur? | What do you believe that it means about your future or your past? | | Is my belief a fact or an opinion? What is the evidence for and against this being true? | | Name your feelings now: how strong are they on a scale of 0-10? |
| Why do you believe it happened? | | | Does my belief help me or keep me feeling negatively? If I was being kind to myself, what could I say differently to myself? | | |

Fertility Related Thought Record – Example

| Trigger situation relating to my fertility | Unhelpful thoughts or beliefs that were prompted... And what I wanted to do when I felt this way... | Describe the feelings you had because of this | Self-compassionate alternatives to thoughts or beliefs that were triggered | What can I do differently in this situation, if not now, in the future? | How do I feel now? Take a breath and notice where you connect to this feeling in your body. Now, rate the intensity of the feeling. |
|---|---|---|---|---|---|
| At a friend's baby shower. | I shouldn't have to do this. | Angry (7). | I can choose to be here or not. She is my best friend so I'll stay for an hour and then arrange to leave. I can challenge myself but don't need to overwhelm myself. | Let Vicky know that I am really happy for her but also finding today challenging and let her know I will be leaving after lunch. She is always understanding about me going through this. | No longer feel nauseous in my tummy and the tightness in my chest has eased (4). |
| | They are all so insensitive talking about babies when I'm going through so much. | Anxious (8). | They don't know what I am going through so they won't know that it is hurtful, and it's normal to want to talk about babies here. I will breathe and go and join my friend and ask about her new job. | Ask John to collect me so I don't need to take public transport alone when I'm feeling like this. We can arrange to go and do something together. There is that film I wanted to see. | I feel sad but not tearful (4). |
| | It's hopeless, it's never going to work for us. They all have it so easy. | Tearful (8). | I am taking a snapshot of my friends' lives. I know they have joyful and challenging times as I do. It is difficult now, but it won't last forever. | Find some space in the garden and do some mindful breathing. | Feeling calmer (6). |
| | John should leave me, he'd be better off. | Feel sick in the stomach. | John loves me and I love him. We are going through this together and need to support each other. | Actually, three of our friends are busy getting things ready. I can get involved with that and it will distract me for a while. | Happy for Vicky (2). |
| | My friends have it so easy, they should stop complaining about their problems. | | | | |

**Journal Activity: Understanding your Thinking Style** 🖊

When you have completed several thought records, you may begin to recognize a pattern of behaviour and thinking emerging. You can deepen your learning and ability to try out new things by writing about your experience.

* How did you find completing your thought record? Did it feel like homework or home learning? Did you resist or engage fully with the exercise?
* Could you find an alternative perspective on your thinking?
* Could you contradict unhelpful beliefs or thoughts against yourself or another?
* When you increased balanced or solution-focused thinking, how did it impact on how you felt?
* Did you notice that it's sometimes easier to engage with self-critical thoughts in times of stress but harder to generate more self-compassionate ones?
* As you evaluate your thought records, what patterns have you noticed?
* What changes in behaviours or what you do can you now experiment with? For example, 'Go out with friends at least once a week even though I want to isolate myself.'
* How will this help you moving forward?

Filling out thought records during times of stress can help you to check-in with what you are saying and doing to help or deepen your emotional experience. You begin to flex the solution-focused and creative part of your mind to increase positive feelings leading to more self-fulfilment.

## Use Positive Self-statements

It is also helpful to combine thought records with positive self-statements to support you on your fertility journey, whether you are trying to conceive naturally or going through assisted fertility treatment. No one ever ran a marathon by telling themselves off at the starting line! How we speak to ourselves is crucial in building self-confidence and kindness which will help you to feel more empowered in any lifestyle choices you make. It is easier to make positive changes if your mind and body are in sync.

Try integrating some positive self-statements, especially during times of challenge when facing fertility-related issues:

- 'We are doing all we can to support ourselves in our desire to have a baby. We are courageous and I will support myself and my partner in this.'
- 'I have gone through similar tests and have managed these. My fears are thoughts not facts; I am strong and can manage this test.'
- 'Keep going (for example, taking medication or injections, etc.) This is only temporary and it is worth it. This short-term discomfort is for my longer-term goal.'
- 'I am a worthwhile person and can show kindness to myself during this time.'

- 'I can bring balance to my feelings and my thoughts and support myself with wise decisions.'
- 'I am a strong woman/man and my life is of value. I can speak to myself in a caring and compassionate way.'
- 'Resisting is not my friend. I can breathe and accept myself fully in this moment and bring myself the kindness of a good and loving friend.'
- 'Well done! I have faced a fearful experience and managed it. I will reward myself with a nurturing event or act of kindness (for example, buy myself some flowers on the way home from my first appointment with a fertility consultant, etc.).'

Now prepare some of your own positive self-statements and write them on brightly coloured card to carry with you to your next appointment, whether that is with your doctor or natural-health practitioner ... or if you are attending a family gathering and need to be armed with the right answers!

### Keep a Gratitude Log

You can also improve how you feel by taking a wider helicopter view of your overall life. It is easy to become micro-focused on the demands and efforts of trying to conceive. When you begin to focus your attention on the areas of your life that contribute positively to you and your relationship, you will increase your sense of gratitude. This naturally contributes towards feelings of appreciation and contentment.

Five Tips for Writing your Gratitude Log:

1. Are there any people you have met during this experience that have helped you?
   'I am grateful to . . . because she/he . . .'
2. When you notice one small thing today that you are grateful for, note it . . . For example, 'I am grateful that the clinic now has green tea and also decaf coffee!'
3. Expand on why you are grateful: 'I am grateful for my husband as he is showing me such kindness and I realize how much he cares.'
4. Don't include the negative! It is easy to sway back into the negative but remember this is a positive log.
5. Keep it simple and be creative. You can put anything in your gratitude log, from noticing birdsong to going to your favourite concert (and put the photo of you in the front row in your gratitude journal).

## Bringing Mindfulness to your Thoughts

Instead of becoming preoccupied with what our thoughts are telling us, we can also become more aware of our thinking with mindfulness. The Buddhist monks refer to the 'monkey mind' as a way to describe the ever-changing busy nature of our mind. I think of busy-mind thoughts as ping-pong balls – bouncing in and out of our mind quickly and, of course, the more anxious we become, the more ping-pong ball thoughts are present.

When you experience fertility-related stress, your mind can become very busy indeed. Even worse, those thoughts are frequently thoughts of regret about the past or creating fearful thoughts about the future. Of course, it is important to plan and aim for goals. However, when our mind becomes preoccupied with every aspect of the present and future, we are trying too hard to influence things that are usually outside of our control, and this in itself leads to more stress.

We can choose to become more aware of our thoughts as mental activity and begin to just notice them – coming and going, ever-changing, from moment to moment. In doing this, we become more present to our experience – not judging it in the moment whether it is good or bad. Though we may be planning for the future, we are not lost in the future while doing it! We become more of a human being than a human doing. We give our attention to the present moment by bringing intentional awareness to our senses; becoming more connected to what we see, hear, smell, taste and feel, rather than what we 'think' about the experience. For example, if you are fearful when going for treatment, you notice the fear – where it sits – and observe it rather than respond to it. You don't become your thoughts of fear but rather notice how you feel it. The feeling then passes more easily as you are not resisting, interpreting it or trying to change it. This approach can also be taken to decision-making around fertility. If you are transitioning from a natural-health approach to assisted reproductive medicine, or a combination of both, you may find that this is also associated with strong feelings or thoughts. Noticing how they manifest in your body in a more observational way allows you to sit with them and not make knee-jerk decisions. It is like being a witness to your thoughts and feelings, as though looking out of the window of a train: you notice how the thoughts rise and fall, judge and evaluate, plan and strate-gize, and may even echo the beliefs of others. Observing them pass by and the sensations that go with them can help you to be more honest to your needs and brings a more gentle clarity to your decision-making.

Mindfulness allows you to begin to notice whatever is present in your mind (thoughts), your body (feelings and sensations) and the sounds and sights that surround you. Rather than becoming swept away with thoughts and inner stories about what you are experiencing, for example, 'This is absolutely awful, I can't cope with doing another test', you are able to observe the fear, without being swept away emotionally by it, observing the thoughts as just that: thoughts not truths. This leads to a greater inner calm-ness and clarity of mind.

## Mindfulness Sitting Meditation

We can easily get caught up in the busyness of our day-to-day living or get trapped in overthinking relationships we are in and challenges that we face . . . what next, what happened, what do I need to change? This 'survival' thinking increases the potential for too much forward planning, living in regrets or worrying about the future. Allowing time to meditate and bring attention back to our breath can help us to anchor more fully in the pres-ent moment. This, in turn, allows a more expansive perspective in regards to our situations and creates more space for a deeper awareness beyond our mental chatter.

Often when caught in mind stories, we breathe in a shallow restricted way, usually in the chest area, and potentially feel quite disconnected. Remember, the mind is only one aspect of us. Expanding the breath helps us to expand our mind awareness leading to a deeper connection with our intuitive, creative, felt sense.

Create a clear space to meditate in at a time when you are less likely to be disturbed or distracted by your surroundings. Many people do sitting meditation at the beginning and end of each day.

- Sitting or kneeling in a comfortable and upright position with your eyes closed (or slightly closed if more comfortable), begin to move your attention towards your inner self.
- Take a few moments to sit in stillness, taking 3 natural deep breaths in and allow your body to let go fully on the out-breath. Notice the rise and fall of your body occurring naturally with each breath.
- Now begin to give focused attention to the movement of your breath. Notice how it enters the nostrils and travels down your body, gently rising in the abdominal area. As you let go, focus on the movement of your breath as it leaves your body.
- Pay close attention to the sensation of the in- and out-breaths, the rising and falling, filling your body and releasing from your body.
- Try not to control the pacing of the breath, just continue to bring your focused attention to the gentle ebb and flow of the breath.
- Allow the silence to expand as you become one with the 'inhale' and 'exhale', living in this moment.
- Notice the urge to be drawn towards your thoughts and mental stories. Notice any judgement present, perhaps

self-judgement for allowing yourself this time. Just notice the urge to go with this wandering mind and gently take your attention back to the breath – filling your body on the in-breath and releasing on the out-breath. Just notice any internal thoughts and let them be, taking your attention back to the breath, anchoring you in the present moment.

- Also acknowledge any feelings or sensations that may arise within and notice any sounds in your environment, as they come closer or move further into the distance. Simply notice these feelings and sensations and take your attention back to your breath. They are in your awareness without being the centre of your attention. Centre yourself back on your moment-to-moment experience, the rising in- and falling out-breath.

- At times you may find that you have become lost in thoughts or feelings. Simply accept that this is a normal part of your mind, to be busy and distracting. Acknowledge this and regain your attention back to the breath and your here-and-now moment.

- Continue to breathe with this natural rhythm for 15–20 minutes and, as you move your attention away from your dedicated meditation time and back to your daily activities, bring this remembered wellness into your day.

Ideally, you would dedicate 15–20 minutes in the morning and evening every day to connect with your meditation practice, in order to reveal how you are in your present and bring balance to your mind and body. Bringing awareness to the present moment, over and over, opens the potential for greater awareness and increased self-kindness.

Incorporating these practical mindfulness-based tools into your daily life will improve communication, support you when dealing with challenging situations, enhance your overall quality of life and, most importantly, help you to regain a sense of personal wellness. Because of its gentle approach, you will be surprised how quickly positive feelings of change begin to happen.

Another area where change can bring benefit quickly is when we manage our relationships with healthier communication styles. This is particularly important as you are likely to engage with many professionals when considering your fertility treatment. When this is balanced with self-nurturing activities, you are likely to have far more enriching interactions.

# CHAPTER 8

## *Self-care and Effective Communication*

........................................

Then it is only kindness
that makes sense anymore,
only kindness that ties your shoes
and sends you out into the day
to mail letters and purchase bread,
only kindness that raises its head
from the crowd of the world to say
It is I you have been looking for,
and then goes with you everywhere
like a shadow or a friend.
EXCERPT FROM 'KINDNESS'
BY NAOMI SHIHAB NYE

........................................

All positive actions begin with a well-meaning intention, which means that we can begin cultivating self-care at any moment by making a decision to do so. Being centred on oneself is often confused with being self-centred, and many of us have been conditioned to believe that giving unconditionally, without question, is the most admirable way to live. While it is important to contribute value in our lives and the lives of others – and research shows that it supports a sense of well-being – it is also important to consider our own needs and learn how to take care of these. This is particularly true during times of emotional strain. Otherwise, it is like collecting water from a well, sharing all the contents with others and not drinking from our own cup. We cannot draw from an empty well!

We can all accept that when we were younger we needed love, affection, care and encouragement, yet as adults we often forget that these same needs still exist. It is particularly important on your fertility journey to empower yourself in the 'now' by taking small compassionate steps towards self-nurture.

## Have the Confidence to Say 'No'

Adopting a positive attitude to life's challenges will lead to a more balanced internal emotional experience, which may include creating space and learning to say 'no' to leave you with more independence to live your own life. We can often become so wrapped up in other people's needs and wants for us, saying 'yes' to their every request, that we have little control over our own time and wants. This is especially true if we are busy 'self-downing' – being mean to ourselves because of the problems we are facing, for example, 'It's typical and no surprise that the problem lies with me.' If we assert no control over other people's demands and requests, it could mean inviting additional stress into our lives at a time when we need to be more self-considered, like organizing to take care of a friend when we are approaching fertility treatment for an embryo transfer. Rather than helping the other person, constant people pleasing can lead to a build-up of secret and unexpressed resentments. Eventually this becomes damaging to our mood and our relationships. It can also mean not following through on a self-care mind–body plan to support emotional and physical well-being because we are busy meeting the endless needs of others.

Often we believe that saying 'no' is rude or invites conflict and, while it's true that many of those benefitting from our constant 'yes' responses may feel conflicted with our 'no' response, we do have a right to consider ourselves in requests on our time and resources. Our needs are equally as important as others' and it is not a form of rejection to become assertive with those needs.

Saying 'no' means:

- You respect your right to say 'no'. You also respect the rights of others to say 'no'.
- You consult with yourself: 'I have consulted with myself and I can/cannot meet with this request.'
- You can say 'no' politely without rejection by expressing it with warmth and in a friendly manner.
- You can express your 'no' without the intention of causing conflict: 'Thank you. However, unfortunately . . .'
- You can choose to say 'yes' if you want to and it works for you too.
- You can be open to further requests, which you will consider on their own merits.
- You can say 'no' in a direct manner, without over-explaining yourself or over-apologizing.
- You can express a 'no' for now without closing the door to a 'yes' in the future, for example meet for a coffee next week instead of today.

- You can express your feelings when saying 'no': 'This is challenging for me.'
- Finally, saying 'no' asserts your right to be treated with respect and to express your own feelings and priorities.

You have the right to get it wrong sometimes and make mistakes as we all do!

## Empower Yourself with Effective Communication

Communicating effectively will usually integrate aspects of assertiveness, sometimes conflict resolution, some empathy and, where possible, unconditional positive regard for yourself and those you wish to communicate with.

You may find yourself being assertive with a colleague at work, but expressing yourself in a passive manner at a meeting with your clinician. Couples and individuals supporting their chance of conception can find themselves meeting with many consultants on their path. Taking the natural-health approach can mean attending fertility consultants including nutritional therapists, fertility counsellors acupuncturists, herbalists and personal trainers. Deciding on the assisted fertility treatment path includes consultations with fertility specialist doctors, nurses, counsellors, embryologists and medical care staff in a hospital or clinical setting.

Many couples and individuals choose an integrative – medical and natural health – approach to enhance their chances of conception, which means they are often attending appointments with practitioners who may or may not endorse each other's views on how to best support your fertility treatment needs.

Learning to communicate assertively to find the most appropriate care will empower you and be beneficial to your overall treatment experience. It also helps you to decide which consultants and treatments are most suitable.

Discussing menstrual cycles, sperm count, semen analysis and ovarian reserve may be commonplace in the daily routine of your fertility consultant. However, it can be a daunting prospect to speak up and effectively assert your own needs in this setting. Communicating assertively in these circumstances can support you in making wise fertility-related treatment choices based on your needs and result in an effective understanding of your consultant's recommendations.

Remember, you have the right to request information and clarification about your fertility health with professionals. Consultants are very used to answering queries relating to fertility health and treatment, even if you feel slightly awkward requesting this information. Asking questions that you think are not medical enough or expressing that you have not understood certain points is perfectly acceptable as the clinician is usually trying to deliver a point for your understanding. By assertively communicating your aspirations and discussing your desired approaches openly, you build on your confidence and this is the key to increasing success. For example, you may want to try acupuncture but do not have the financial resources to attend each week. Communicating this to your therapist assertively will mean you are not increasing stress by engaging in treatment that you cannot financially support. It is more likely to lead to your desired outcome, for example, attending every two or three weeks as arranged. After all, this treatment is to support a reduction in stress! Initially, this will mean stepping outside of your comfort zone as you learn to communicate in a non-threatening, assertive manner, leading to a more self-empowered and confident self.

**Assertive communication assertions:**
- My goals are of value and I count.
- Your goals are of value and you count.

**Aggressive communication assertions:**
- My goals are of value and I count.
- Your goals are of no value and you do not count.

**Passive-aggressive communication assertions:**
- I am of value and I count, but I will not express this. I may communicate it by sulking or quietly punishing you.
- You don't count but I will not communicate this clearly!

**Passive communication assertions:**
- My goals are of no value and I don't count.
- Your goals are of value and you count more than me.

## Examine Your Communication Style

Many of us relate less assertively in professional or medical settings. We may be very confident expressing our needs in intimate relationships but feel less sure of asserting them in a work or professional setting. Consider your behaviour in regards to fertility-related conversations or appointments, especially if you have experienced disappointments or let downs. Think of your most recent significant fertility-related experience and circle your most common communication approaches.

## Passive

Ways of being:

- Victim and feeling like a loser: 'Poor me, bad things always happen to me', 'I'm hopeless at everything.' (This self-pitying approach can mean it takes longer to recover after testing and treatment setbacks.)
- Avoidant and self-downing: 'I don't like this so I will stay away from any similar challenge now and in the future', 'It's all my fault and always is.'

Ways of thinking:

- 'I am hopeless.'
- 'I probably don't deserve it anyway.'
- 'I don't have the right to ask or effect change.'

## Aggressive

Ways of being:

- Demanding: 'My way is always right, not yours!' This will usually close you off from the other person's point of view.

- Blaming, disempowering the other by being overly critical (can translate into blaming partner for the fertility problem).
- Sarcastic, may also use humour to put others down.
- Enlists others against person, for example, character-assassinate individual (the treating consultant, for example) in a blog or speak to colleagues or family about 'totally terrible' person ('Aunty Mary who keeps asking me if I am planning a family!').
- Shouting or aggressively giving orders rather than making requests.
- Using 'should' statements: 'You should do this, you shouldn't do that . . .', 'You said . . . that's a stupid approach', etc.

Ways of thinking:

This generally leads to quite rigid and demanding ways of thinking about others, for example:
- 'How dare they?'
- 'They know nothing.'
- 'They did this deliberately.'
- 'They absolutely shouldn't do this.'

**Passive-aggressive**

Ways of being:

When individuals express themselves in passive-aggressive ways, they can become manipulative rather than confidently asserting their needs. Blaming is usually done indirectly and the individual tends to be reactive and put others down in a very non-direct manner. Overall feelings of resentment and powerlessness are expressed in unhealthy ways, which could include emotional bribery or commonly having judgemental responses. Being passive-aggressive can include the following traits:

- Being a martyr
- Controlling by sulking
- Becoming quiet and withdrawn
- Overexplaining and agreeing to everything in an apologetic manner: 'I'm sorry . . . it doesn't matter . . . don't worry'

Ways of thinking:

This leads to very depleting ways of thinking, such as:

- 'They're inconsiderate'
- 'I hate them for making me do this'
- 'I say I don't mind but they should know that I do'
- 'I always have to do it' (over-generalizing without acknowledging partner's contribution or support)
- 'Nobody considers me'

**Assertive**

Ways of being:

When communicating in an assertive manner, we are more likely to have more of our needs met (though not always) and feel less overall resentment. Needs are expressed with an understanding that the other person has choice in regards to how they may respond. One's own feelings and desires are expressed openly – 'I would like . . .', 'I wonder if we could . . .' – in a clear, decisive and unapologetic manner. In general this leads to happier individuals as they are congruent and honest without being domineering. They tend to take considered risk but do not blame themselves or others if it doesn't work out. They tend to initiate positive action if things are not working out for them.

When we are being assertive, we tend to:

* Listen attentively with an open and relaxed posture
* Take responsibility and be self-empowered
* Be reasonable and more accepting in our decision-making
* Request rather than demand

Ways of thinking:

Being assertive leads to more flexible ways of thinking, for example:

* 'I can ask but it's okay to hear that it's not possible'
* 'I can request but am open to another option'
* 'I can make other choices'
* 'I understand this . . . however I request this . . .'
* 'I understand your perspective but also value mine'

Being assertive in your communication when liaising with medical professionals can be very helpful to provide further clarification or options, for example:

* 'I don't agree with my treatment, your treatment or this approach . . . what are the gains and losses of X over Y?'

It also leads to more solution-focused approaches, such as:

- 'How about . . . ?'
- 'How can we . . . ?'
- 'How do you feel . . . ?'

---

**Journal Activity:**

**Understanding Your Communication Style** 🖊

- How do you express your needs during your natural or assisted fertility support sessions or with your partner? Would you say that you communicate assertively, aggressively, passively or in a passive-aggressive manner?
- Does this approach help or hinder you?
- Can you think of a time that you communicated in a way that you were content with in a challenging situation? Write about what you did and what this felt like.
- Have there been times when you said 'yes' when you really meant 'no'? Write about this, what happened and how you felt.
- What communication goals would you like to establish? What could you do at your next meeting to put this goal into action?

---

Remember that change takes time – take a 'progress not perfection' approach to test driving your new communication style.

## Increase Your Nurturing Activities

We usually don't notice when the scales have been tipped in favour of people, places and things that deplete our energy and resources. However, staying positive and healthy on your fertility journey includes bringing balance back into your life and engaging with experiences that increase your good mood and people that encourage joy and emotional support in your life.

During times of distress, we can often decrease the activities that actually energize us as we become withdrawn and lose interest. This has a spiral effect: the fewer engaging activities we do, the less energy we have and, eventually, this can lead to low mood or depression with associated feelings of exhaustion. Bringing some balance back will begin to restore your energy reserves.

---

**Journal Activity: Nurturing and Depleting Experiences** ✎

Fill out the journal page below and make a note of your usual daily activities by connecting to whether they are energizing or depleting in nature. This could be relating to present-day activities but can also include events in the past.

On the '+' side write down all the things that you enjoy, hobbies past and present and list the people you like to meet with. Also include places that leave you feeling better. You can complete one for a typical weekday and another one for the weekend.

---

On the '−' side, write down all the things that you find challenging, activities that deplete your energy, people you find difficult at the moment and places you would rather not visit.

You may find that some are written in the middle of the page – both elevating and depleting at times.

| + | − |
|---|---|
| I enjoy spending time with ... My friend Kate: she always makes me laugh, cooks great food and doesn't talk incessantly about her children. | I feel depleted when I spend time engaging with ... Aunt Maura, who always asks me when we're going to plan for a baby ... if only she knew! Janet, because she really doesn't get where I'm at right now. |
| I benefit from this hobby or pastime ... I really enjoyed playing the piano but haven't done much of that lately. Going to hear a band. | I find it a chore to ... Talk to everyone about how my treatment is going. Perhaps I need to manage this better for me. |
| I usually feel better after visiting ... ... the coast. ... a coffee shop with my book. | I don't enjoy going to ... ... the clinic − when I hear bad news. |
| What lifts my mood? The clinic − when I hear good news. | What lowers my mood? Work − when colleagues are busy making plans in the canteen for their family. |
| What lowers tension? Work − it's where I do really well and have some distraction from all this process. | What increases stress? Going on too many blogs. When I go on once a week, it's more helpful. |

Doing this exercise can help to draw your attention to areas of your life that you may need to increase to support energy and well-being levels, and other areas that you may need to avoid or limit during this time. Surrounding yourself with encouraging friends and limiting time with friends who don't understand your journey will help you feel supported and give you some necessary 'time out' from the fertility-related world.

Being absorbed in an interesting activity can help to reduce distress and give you some valuable distraction during the waiting times for test results, which can be very stressful. You may wish to take up a new interest or get in touch with an old friend. Having a choice of activities can give you another focus.

Be creative – you may not have the money to book a holiday away to your favourite place, but you could arrange an interesting day out to a free exhibition. Taking up an energizing activity can help to lift your mood while enjoying some relaxing time out can support you to release tension. You could choose from some of the following ideas and, of course, create your own. Enjoy!

Leisure

* Join a book club or read a novel.
* Learn to sing or join a choir.
* Arrange coffee or a dinner party with friends.
* Frame your favourite pictures (include holidays and friends) and put them up around the house, or paint without being self-critical.
* Join the gym or take up restorative yoga – it helps you make friends with your body again.

- Visit an exhibition or go and see a feel-good film at the cinema.
- Arrange an intimate night in for two, complete with sumptuous food and soft lighting.
- Dress up in clothes that make you feel good.
- Have a safe haven room in your home – a fertility-free zone.
- Have intimacy without purpose!
- Join a dance group – choose an energizing form, from ballroom to belly dancing!
- Compile a CD of your favourite or relaxing music – if you're having fertility treatment use these CDs to create a less clinical personal atmosphere. Play some music from a happy time in your life and sing along (loudly!).
- Take up a musical instrument (30 per cent of us have musical instruments in our home but don't play them!).

Out and About

- Go for a walk in nature, on the beach or in a park.
- Visit a place you have never seen.
- Arrange a spontaneous trip with your partner.
- Stroll around a bric-a-brac shop.
- Visit an art gallery.
- Buy a plant or do some gardening.

Self-nurture

- Go to bed early with a good book.
- Buy a candle in your favourite scent or some aromatherapy oils for your bath.

- Try out some body healing: aromatherapy, reflexology, massage, acupuncture.
- Meditate – to centre your body and calm your mind.
- Teach yourself some relaxation techniques: progressive muscle relaxation, mindfulness meditation, creative visualization (for example the safe-place exercise, page 62).
- Write a list of all the things you are grateful for – big and small.
- Write a list of positive things you have done. If you're stuck, dial a friend!

## Mindfulness Loving-Kindness Meditation

The loving-kindness meditation dates back 2,500 years and was first taught by the Buddha to help individuals to overcome fear. Having a deep desire, such as wanting a child, and facing difficulties in relation to this can frequently give rise to waves of fear and feelings of anxiety. Loving-kindness meditation is an antidote to self-criticism, fear and loss.

Increasing self-kindness has also been attributed to bringing more self-acceptance and equanimity. We can also practise loving-kindness towards others, for example our partner, even if we are unable to feel loving thoughts towards them presently. Finally, we can widen our loving-kindness and mindful attention towards an issue we are facing, for example the whole fertility-related problem.

Increasing self-acceptance and kindness does not mean we are giving in to the problem, rather it allows us to be okay with ourselves as we journey through it. In addition to increasing acceptance of where we are in the 'now', whether that is deeply challenging (facing tests and treatment) or experiencing a joyful breakthrough, loving-kindness supports us to be true to ourselves rather than being blown by all the winds of change.

Keep yourself, your partner, a difficult person (perhaps a relative insensitive to your fertility problems!) or your current fertility challenge in mind and send them an intention of loving-kindness, as follows:

- Allow 15 or 20 minutes for this meditation. Sit in a relaxed and upright posture in a calm and supportive environment.
- Spend a few minutes scanning your body from head to toe and noticing any areas of tension. Gently invite yourself to 'drop your shoulders', 'release your jaw', 'let go of tension in your belly', 'let go'.
- Take a deep breath into your tummy area, allowing it to rise with the in-breath and release on the out-breath. There is no need to try and breathe 'right' or to control the breath. Gain a gentle breathing rhythm.
- As you hold yourself, another or a situation in mind for this exercise, you may find that your mind wanders – just notice if this happens and bring your attention back to your intention of loving-kindness.
- Also, notice when these thoughts contain a difficult emotional tone, such as judgement, irritation or despair. Just notice these feelings without trying to move towards them or push them away. Notice that feelings come and go and take your focus back towards an intention of loving-kindness.

- You may find it difficult to feel open to sending love towards yourself or feeling compassion towards a person you have difficulty with. Just notice and recognize this difficulty, without assessing it. Continue to bring your intention back to being open to each of the phrases; towards opening your heart to all the possibilities of self-acceptance and forgiveness.

Hold yourself at the centre of your mind and take a moment to reflect on the following phrases and invite them into your being:

*May I be well*
*May I be happy*
*May I know peace*
*May I be free from suffering*
*May my mind feel well*
*May my body feel well*
*May I live joyfully*
*May I be content*
*May I have gratitude*
*May I feel safe*
*May I be kind*
*May I know love*

Now expand your loving-kindness awareness to those you are grateful for on your fertility journey, and to family and friends who share your process. Holding an image of the individual in your mind, reflect on the following phrases:

*May they be well*
*May they be happy*
*May they know peace*
*May they be free from suffering*
*May they feel well in mind*
*May they feel well in body*
*May they know joy*
*May they feel content*
*May they know gratitude*
*May they feel safe*

Picture some of the neutral people that have crossed your path on this journey; acquaintances and others whom you have met along the way. Sending them loving-kindness, focus on the following phrases:

*May they be safe*
*May they be well in body*
*May they be well in mind*
*May they be free from suffering*
*May they know peace*

Now we bring into mind people or situations that we struggle with. It may be someone who has harmed us emotionally or psychologically. In picturing this person or situation, we bring compassion towards ourselves as we become emotionally less stuck in the negative energy exchange – in our thoughts and feelings – between us and the person we have difficulty with.

We also bring an intention of forgiveness towards the situation, understanding that conflict and unkindness often grow from the seeds of fear and mistrust. This meditation cultivates empathy – the capacity to walk in a person's shoes and better understand their story and their way of being. Be gentle with yourself with this loving-kindness meditation and keep in mind that we bring our attention to those situations and people that we find challenging rather than focusing on those that we feel overwhelmed by (this is more suited to therapeutic work with a mental-health practitioner, for example a fertility counsellor, psychotherapist or psychologist).

Gently and with loving-kindness towards yourself, expand this to those you have difficulty with:

*May they be healthy in mind*
*May they be healthy in body*
*May this person be safe*
*May they know peace*
*May they live with ease*

Finally, we expand our attention to the wider community and all living beings without limitation. To all those you know and do not know:

*May all living beings be safe*
*May all living beings know peace*
*May all living beings know joy*
*May all living beings live with ease*
*May all living beings live with comfort*
*May all living beings know love*
*May all living beings know kindness*

### Journal Activity: Trying for a Baby ✎

- Write about your experience of trying for a baby.
- What are your deepest thoughts about yourself and any areas of difficulty relating to this?
- What are your deepest thoughts about your partner and any difficulties you have both experienced?
- What are the feelings that arise from these thoughts?
- Bring an intention of inner healing towards these thoughts and feelings in the loving-kindness meditation.

Cultivating loving kindness can bring a welcome closeness back into your relationships, as can fostering deeper listening and paying attention to your needs and those of your partner, as expressed in the next chapter.

# CHAPTER 9

## *Caring for Your Relationship and Understanding Each Other*

Never look back unless you are planning to go that way.

HENRY DAVID THOREAU

All relationships face challenging times and it can be difficult to know how to look after your own emotional needs when faced with trying for a baby, much less the needs of your relationship and those of your partner. However, shining a light on areas where the relationship may have become stuck and working towards communicating with each other in an empathic and positive way, can support you both in connecting at a deeper level, which naturally helps you to successfully navigate difficulties together. Of course, it is necessary to sometimes reflect on our past and how we developed our beliefs and relationship patterns to learn new approaches. However, the quotation above is also true insofar as it is important that we do not get stuck in overthinking our past experiences or perceived mistakes.

There are significant life goals that tend to draw couples together or cause relationship problems, and how we express and respond to these life events is crucial to the overall health of the relationship. The desire to have a child is one of those life goals, as are: where you want to live; how you relate to each other intimately; what your financial goals are; and what ambitions you both share. These shared values either contribute to the building and security of a relationship or tear it down from within. When you are both journeying towards shared aspirations it is easier to enjoy the relationship after the initial fireworks have dwindled, as there are strong foundations to build a lasting, secure and nurturing relationship and keep the flames of romance burning.

As you are both individuals and also part of a couple, you will naturally approach these life goals in different but ideally compatible ways, relying on a healthy dialogue and sometimes compromising your individual 'right way' for the overall good of the relationship. When one of these important life goals is blocked, for example, trying for a baby, it can lead to powerful emotional responses which can bring pressure and conflict to the relationship at a time when both individuals need more understanding. Men can feel that they are required to perform as they need to produce sperm samples and have them graded for quality, and women can feel resentful at having to be the one that misses so much time off work and make so many life changes to support their fertility health, or spend their evenings administering injections. This can be accompanied by financial insecurity as some couples take out loans or spend their life savings to invest in their fertility treatment. Holidays and other nurturing activities may also need to be put on hold.

Often I meet couples who describe feeling much closer despite having experienced fertility problems and this supports their relationship long after treatment. They have learned a resilience that has involved listening to and empathizing with each other, in addition to expressing caring behaviours towards each other and taking mutual responsibility in times of need, and beyond.

By understanding our communication styles, how we learned them and also how to change them if we need to, we can learn to grow and feel safe enough to express our needs at an emotional level and also to reflect this to our significant other. How we communicate during these times can either see us through and lead to a stronger relationship or create the potential to cause deeper hurts. You may wish to consider doing the following exercises with the support of a therapist.

## Understanding Your Communication Style

The intuitive mind is a sacred gift and the rational mind is a faithful servant. We have created a society that honours the servant and has forgotten the gift.

Tom Culham, *Ethics Education of Business Leaders* (2013)

I know you've heard it before but it's true what they say: our childhood and early life experiences and relationships influence how we respond in our current relationship. How we observed our parents or carers relating and the messages that we received can manifest to either help or hinder our communication styles with our chosen partner. If you had a nurturing early childhood environment, where you were encouraged to trust and share your intuitive feelings and to develop independent thinking while also being considerate of others, you are more likely to encourage and mirror these qualities in your relationship. However, if emotional nurturing was lacking, you can become disconnected from your thinking or feeling energy. This is because early life messages encouraged our 'survival' brain to become over-activated, causing us to react with fight, freeze or flee. These remembered, although not always consciously experienced, feelings or sensations can get triggered easily and we are more likely to react from our remembered sense of danger with repeated fight, freeze or flee patterns. Reducing the need to have the 'survival' part of our brain activated, for example being hypervigilant in times of danger (e.g. in response to an angry caregiver approaching), allows for space to be creative in our problem-solving and to relate in an emotionally safe way.

Take some time to write about your early life or first relationship experiences. This will help you to explore your cognitive, emotional and behavioural blueprint. Remember, this can bring up some challenging feelings so check-in with yourself and take breaks, only writing as deeply or as little as you need to. This is about supporting you to integrate healthy communication styles in your present relationship and not about deepening old wounds.

Aim to do the following journaling exercises over a number of days or even weeks rather than in one sitting. Allow your learning to unfold in the spirit of positive self-reflection and enquiry. This will help you to focus on what is working in addition to what you would like to see change in yourself and also in your relationship.

Notice what comes up for you individually and as a couple and aim to explore your findings with acceptance and understanding rather than judgement and self-criticism. These exercises are aimed at deepening compassion towards yourself and your partner and connecting with your shared hopes moving forward.

---

**Journal Activity** 🖊

Understanding Your Relational Blueprint

Take some time to write about and understand your logical mind and how past learning may be influencing the present.

* As a child or young person, were you encouraged to think for yourself: 'That's a good idea, and how might you do that?', 'That's very clever, I'm really proud of you' – or was your thinking expression suppressed – 'That's really stupid, how could you think that?', 'That makes no sense at all'?
* Were you listened to and encouraged to express yourself or were you talked over and ignored? For example, 'Don't be a nuisance', 'I'm busy now, come back later.'
* Were your ideas encouraged to flow freely or were they quashed before they started?

---

Now think about your relationship with your partner:

- How do you encourage your partner to think for themselves or do you think for yourself in your relationship?
- Do you have a voice in the relationship or do you suppress your needs and aim to please?
- How do you express your needs, wants and desires? In a controlled or controlling way or a live-and-let-live way?

## Understanding Your Behavioural Blueprint

Think about your early life or initial relationship experiences. What messages did you receive about doing or behaving?

- Did you learn to trust in your own ability even if you made a mistake – 'It's about participating but not always winning, well done' – or did you learn that every mistake is a failure: 'You can't do anything right. How did others in your class do?', 'I'll do that, it's really not done properly at all'?
- Did you receive messages that people are trustworthy or untrustworthy?
- Were you encouraged to have a balance between doing and being: to work towards goals and also to relax, play and have fun?
- What are your positive memories about your childhood? How do they make you feel?

Now think about your relationship with your partner:

* How are the mistakes or disappointments that you experience in the relationship and in your life together treated?
* What beliefs do you hold about things that don't always work out? Do you generally perceive it as:
    * 'It is as it is; that can happen sometimes';
    * 'I tried the best that I could and I need to take care of myself after experiencing that loss';
    * Or do you hold self-negating beliefs: 'This means I'm a failure', 'This means I am not loveable', or 'Bad things always happen to me/us'?
    * Are there similarities with your past? And past beliefs in similar situations?
* Do you trust others to support you and do you choose trustworthy and empathic relationships? Or are you in a 'differentiated' relationship; physically sharing the same space but not working towards things together?
* Do you both enjoy fun times and relaxation in addition to working towards mutual goals?
* What are the positive qualities about your relationship? How do they make you feel?

Understanding Your Feelings

Take some time to remember your experience of being nurtured and held, and how feelings were cared for in your early life relationships.

- Were you encouraged to trust and express your feelings, for example, 'I'm sorry you feel that, come and have a hug'? Or were feelings minimized or discouraged, for example, 'You're way too over-sensitive' or 'You're a boy, stop crying'?
- Were you or someone in your family rewarded for having no regulation with emotions, for example, was your mother, sister, brother or yourself given lots of positive or negative focus of attention for being regularly upset or angry? Were they a victim or a persecutor? In these instances the message can be that behaving in this way will gain attention. This can lead to a learned helplessness. It can also encourage a belief that other people's needs are more important than yours and that you should not express your own needs in favour of constantly taking care of those of others.

Now think about your relationship and explore how you both express your feelings:

- Do you/does your partner listen and empathize when you/he/she expresses their emotional needs or are they ignored? Can you or your partner hear your emotional needs in times of distress? Do you both really listen to each other?
- Are feelings given space in the relationship or is there an unwritten rule: no feelings, as expressing feelings means being out of control?
- Are healthy negative and positive feelings nurtured in the relationship?

- Is there equal space given for feelings in the relationship or does one partner demand more space for their feelings at the cost of another?
- Can your relationship hold and support healthy negative emotions such as sadness, loss, healthy anger, hurt and grief?
- Can your relationship hold healthy boundaries when unhealthy negative emotions, such as unhealthy anger (blaming, over-generalizing, etc.), unhealthy envy ('It's your fault'), guilt, shaming or unhealthy jealousy, are being overly expressed?

## Adjusting Your Communication Style

When we change how we automatically react to our own or perceived shortcomings in our partner to more empathic ways of communicating, we release the relationship from toxic communication patterns. This energizes the relationship and provides equal space for both partners to express their needs, wants and desires. In so doing, you reignite your relationship with the love and caring attention that you both enjoyed in its early stages. Connecting at a heartfelt level helps you both to navigate your fertility journey more easily. It leads to more communication flow and less defensiveness towards each other. Our hearts can be open when we don't feel the need to constantly defend ourselves.

Behavioural change is never easy; otherwise there wouldn't be an ongoing multibillion-pound dieting industry! It requires patience and determination to instigate small changes in behaviour, coupled with an understanding of why it is no longer healthy to continue to communicate in an unhealthy way. How we communicate our need for change to our partner and in our relationship is also important, if we want lasting change to happen.

How do you express difficult feelings, such as frustration or anger? Is it similar or different to observed behaviour in your family of origin? Recognizing your own 'blueprint' can help you to establish a different way of communicating in times of distress or emotional need. You will no longer automatically react to negative pre-learned beliefs about yourself, others and the world. Equally, you will no longer enable others to maintain their negative pre-learned beliefs and behaviours in your relationship with them.

Each partner may wish to explore the questions above, over a two-week period, to gain a sense of their own 'blueprint' and then take 45 minutes to write about their healthy emotional needs by exploring and expressing the following:

## Journal Activity

- What do I need in times of distress that I may not have received in my early life experiences?
- How could I help myself with this? For example, what nurturing activities do I need at that time and what do I not need?
- How could I request that my partner help me with this?
- How may this help the way I feel?

- What do I do when I feel these needs are not being met? What healthy and unhealthy reactions do I usually have when my needs are not being met? How could I change these?
- What request do I have of my partner to help support this positive change?
- What strengths do I have even in times of distress?
- What strengths does my partner have even in times of distress?
- What are the positive qualities in the relationship that we can and do build on?
- What would I hope to see done differently?
- What kind of relationship would I like to move towards – in the good times and also in the challenging times?

## Using Active Listening

Now take 20 minutes each to express what you have learned. This involves 'actively' listening to the other: listening with your whole attention – your eyes, ears and body posture listening to your partner and vice versa. Remember, this exercise is not about fixing anything for your partner. As the 'active listener', you listen rather than interrupt or make suggestions. It is also not about pointing out or expanding on the shortcomings you perceive in your partner. This would cause deeper hurt rather than being a healing experience of self-exploration.

Active listening is about understanding at a deeper level what it is like for the other person when they are feeling distressed and how we may be present to them, while also being present to our own needs. Many old wounds and frustrations can begin to heal if we truly listen and empathize with the emotional needs of our partner while also respecting our own needs. It brings more gentle awareness and kindness into the relationship. By truly listening to what it is like to walk in our partner's shoes, we can begin to feel a deeper sense of empathic understanding and connection towards them and ourselves. This deeper connection can also open the relationship to new intimacies of mind and body.

## Conflict Resolution

When you resolve conflicts with respect, your relationship becomes stronger. Blame and demands are replaced with taking responsibility for your own part in the conflict and, rather than arguing and demanding that your partner changes, you request change where you see an issue. In this way the real issues are resolved rather than power games played out, further undermining the relationship.

In conflict resolution, you do not lose sight of your partner's needs in your desire to have your own met. Your partner remains the person you love rather than an opponent who needs to be corrected! And sometimes, you agree to disagree.

Firstly, identify your need. Arguments are usually about expressing our frustrations, but behind the frustration is usually a 'need' that is not being met. This has usually been simmering for quite some time before the emotional outburst! Recognizing your feelings sooner helps to release the tension behind them. For example, if you feel that your partner is not taking the fertility issue seriously – perhaps they are drinking and smoking in the lead up to taking some important fertility-related tests or samples – rather than wait until this feels unbearable, express how you feel, what you would like to see change and also try to gain some understanding about how they may be feeling and thinking in response to the upcoming tests. This approach is more likely to be inclusive and elicit positive change, rather than a confrontational once.

Taking a conflict-resolution approach to differences allows you to seek a solution where the needs of both you and your partner are given equal importance. It is important to take a wider perspective – understanding that there are two different but equally valid views of the problem. Viewing your conflicts in this way allows both parties to win rather than believing that, 'My way is right and you should do it my way', usually accompanied by an unhealthy expression of, 'I'm right, you're wrong' anger.

### Top Tips for Resolving Conflict

- Wait until the very strong emotion has subsided somewhat, then ask yourself: 'What would I like to see change?'
- Understand your motivation: 'Why do I want this to change? What is my underlying need?'
- Take a helicopter view: 'Am I open to seeing and understanding that my partner has another point of view and it is just as valid as mine?'
- Gain perspectives: 'How can we share our beliefs, thoughts and attitudes about this?'
- Keep focused: 'How can I express this by dealing with the issue and expressing my need, rather than finding fault or attacking the other person?' Avoid statements such as, 'You always do this', 'You are so selfish' as these can lead to

over-generalizing and overestimating the intentions behind the action.

Try using the following dialogue or similar when you are expressing your request for change:

When you do . . .          (name the frustration)
I feel . . .               (name and own your own feeling)
I would like it/prefer it
if you could . . .         (your request of your partner)

Example:
When you ask me if I have taken my fertility supplements each day.
I feel undermined and mistrusted, and this leads to me feeling agitated.
I'm asking that you refrain from asking me this every day, even though I understand you mean well. I'm asking you to trust that I want this as much as you do even if I do miss the occasional supplement.

Use phrasing such as 'I am . . .' or 'I feel . . .', rather than 'You make me feel . . .': no one can 'make' you feel a certain way. When your buttons are pressed, you choose your response. And remember a request is not a demand!

## Mindfulness RAIN Meditation

If you are overwhelmed by difficult emotions, such as anger, fear or a sense of hopelessness, and don't yet feel ready to express your needs in a balanced and considered way to your partner, you may benefit from a mindfulness exercise called 'RAIN', first expounded by the mindfulness teacher and author, Tara Brach:[1]

**Recognize** what is happening within.

**Allow** things to be as they are in this present moment. Gently encourage yourself to allow rather than resist feelings, thoughts and sensations: 'It is as it is . . . let it be.' Say yes to the part of you resisting things as they are in this present moment. Say yes to the part of you saying 'I do not want this.' Open yourself to how you are right now. You are noticing things as they are in this moment, rather than judging it or trying to push any feelings, thoughts or sensations away or bringing them towards you.

**Investigate** this inner experience with close attention. How am I now, on a feeling, thinking and sensing level? What is happening for me in this moment? What is calling for my attention? Notice what type of thoughts you are having. Just note them rather than engage with or embellish them. What feelings are most present? Where do I feel these feelings and thoughts in my body? Is it pleasant or unpleasant? If it is uncomfortable, like anger, guilt, sadness or fear, how do I feel it? Do I experience a tightness or heaviness? Where do I notice these feelings are held in my body? Can I feel the experience as a whole – in my mind and my body and in my emotional centre – the heart? How can I bring kindness to myself and the situation? What most needs my acceptance?

You may wish to ask yourself the following questions:

- What do you believe? Do you believe you are failing or that you will not cope in the future? Do you believe that your relationship will not cope in the future?

- Where does this belief express itself in your body? Really pay attention to how you feel in response to your beliefs.
- What sensations do you hold in your body? Is your body tight and restricted or relaxed? Just notice the sensations and where they are most present.

Now ask your most challenged part of you: what do you want from me? What do you need? Do you need to be accepted, cared for, forgiven and loved unconditionally? Your needs may come to you with intuitive words, an image or a desire to be held. Notice your needs and how they express themselves.

**Non-identification.** As you become present with unconditional positive regard towards your inner experience, an expansive awareness begins to hold your thoughts, feelings and sensations – a whole mind–body experience being held with gentle acceptance. This expansive space has room to allow your sensations, thoughts and feelings to come and go, in and out of your awareness. You no longer identify with the painful emotion or difficulty. You are no longer swept away by thoughts or feelings. Instead you hold it all in a gentle, spacious awareness.

Generating this type of self and body awareness means you are not controlled by the events happening around you. RAIN meditation can help to foster increased feelings of self-kindness and inner calm. You are less likely to find yourself ruminating with fertility-related thoughts and more likely to welcome more head space and peace of mind. Enjoy inviting more unconditional self-compassion towards yourself.

## Caring Activities

Combining a deeper understanding of ourselves and engaging with the hard work of changing our behaviours – not automatically reacting from old learning but putting into practice new learning (progress not perfection!) – is helped by increasing caring activities to nurture our relationship. It is not uncommon to begin to forego the pleasures of shared time together in favour of investing more time in areas that may have been missed due to meeting the demands of all those extra fertility-related appointments. For example, you may increasingly work later to make up for lost time in the office and so time out together can get missed. Making an appointment with each other can easily be dropped down the priority list and, consequently, one or both individuals begin to feel uncared for by their partner. Hidden resentments can begin to surface with each individual chastising themselves or each other for not being worthy of love, as the caring side of the relationship continues to dwindle.

Research shows that our own happiness increases when we give to others while also caring for ourselves.[2] This expresses a 'You are worthy of attention' and 'I am worthy of attention' belief that is both nurturing and giving and may require that we step outside of our comfort zone. By practising kindness towards others, our own happiness increases and this naturally has a positive and energizing effect on our relationship.

Caring actions can be based on what you receive now and would like to receive more of, or you can draw inspiration from remembering the things you enjoyed when you first began dating or at a particularly good time in your relationship. Using the table below for guidance, write down a list of caring activities that your partner does that you enjoy, enjoyed or would like to enjoy moving forward and pass them to each other. Write spontaneously for 10 minutes and then swap lists. Come to an agreement about what is a reasonable number of caring behavioural 'gifts' you can give each other on a daily and weekly basis.

| Caring behaviours in our relationship | What positive feelings do you have when you receive these caring 'gifts'? |
| --- | --- |
| Things you enjoy that your partner does for you . . . | |
| Things that you enjoyed in the past that your partner did for you . . . | |
| Things that you would like your partner to do more of . . . | |

For example:

| Caring behaviours in our relationship | What positive feelings do you have when you receive these caring 'gifts'? |
|---|---|
| **Things you enjoy that your partner does for you . . .** <br> *Brings me coffee in the morning* <br> *Drives me to the train station.* | *I feel looked after.* <br> *I feel valued.* |
| **Things that you enjoyed in the past that your partner did for you . . .** <br> *Loved it when you surprised me with planned nights out, for example buying theatre and concert tickets in our first years together.* <br> *When you used to occasionally buy me flowers.* | *I loved those 'date' nights with elements of surprise. They felt exciting. I would love more 'date' nights, even though I know we don't have as much money at the moment. Perhaps we could go on 'budget' fun nights out together again.* |
| **Things that you would like your partner to do more of . . .** <br> *Random surprises that show you care and have affection for us even in this difficult time.* | *It makes me feel cherished and important to you.* |

## Healing Touch

When regaining aspects of intimacy in your relationship, you can also draw on the healing power of touch. Our overall well-being is enhanced when we feel the relaxed and nurturing physical presence of our partner. This can often be the first part of the relationship to be withdrawn when either partner is experiencing stress or undertaking ongoing physical examinations. Many people describe a feeling of disconnect from their body as it no longer feels their own – not doing what they want it to do (get pregnant) and experiencing fertility tests and treatment. This can become mentally and physically exhausting, and healing touch can bring some much-needed energy flow back to your body, contributing to a sense of physical balance. A balanced body also helps to balance the mind.

### Massage

Giving and receiving a massage from your partner can bring pleasure and closeness back into the relationship. When giving your partner a massage:

+ Do it at a time when you feel energized yourself as you will then freely give love and care in a well-meaning way.

* **Please note:** do not undertake these massage treatments if you or your partner has any medical conditions that are contraindicated to do so. This can include having previously experienced deep-vein thrombosis, any spinal injury or heart problems. If you have any concerns, check with your medical consultant first.

- Wear loose clothing and ensure you are both in a comfortable position before you start.
- Combine the massage with some relaxation music, aromatherapy oils (four drops of lavender oil in an oil burner will fill the air with relaxing aromas) or candles, and soft lighting so that all the senses can benefit.
- Switch off your mobile phones and electronic devices as they do not contribute to your couple's sanctuary!
- Don't keep checking in with your partner asking questions such as, 'Are you enjoying this?' or 'Is that enough?' as this will prevent them from relaxing deeply into the massage.
- Ensure that you have a yoga mat, blanket, pillow and a glass of water as required.
- Buy some organic massage oil from a good health store. Good massage oils include grape seed or almond oils.

When receiving a massage from your partner:

- Agree in advance how much pressure you would like during your massage and indicate the areas of tension that you would like your partner to focus on.
- Trust that your partner wants to give you the massage and that he/she will take care of you during this healing time together.
- Doing yoga breaths – deeply breathing in through your nose and releasing out through your mouth – will help to calm the nervous system.
- If your mind is busy, just notice the thoughts and don't enter into their content. As you breathe in, repeat the word 'calm' in your mind and as you breathe out, repeat the words 'letting go'.

Heart Opening Exercise

This heart opening exercise encourages closeness by giving and receiving touch grounded in breath, openness and compassion. It helps to bring you closer, builds trust and releases tension before you move into more stress-releasing body massage.

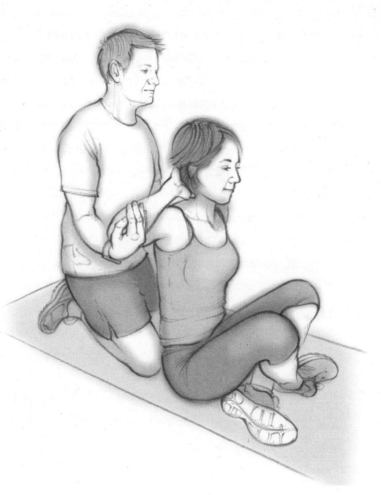

Heart Opening Exercise

The giver is kneeling with legs apart behind the receiver on a yoga mat or blanket. The receiver is leaning slightly back on the giver. Legs are crossed and slightly apart, resting on the mat with the giver's legs resting on the outside of the receiver's legs.

**Receiver:** place your arms behind your head and relax your head by leaning it against your interlaced hands. Feel the stretch in your chest as you bring a deep breath in through your nostrils.

**Giver:** place your arms under your partner's armpits with your hands holding back his/her elbow area. Push your body gently against his/her torso as you do this. Slide your arms up further so that you are holding and stretching his/her forearms and opening their chest with your support. Hold this position for 8 breaths together.

Following this, the receiver moves gently into lying face down on the mat, turning their head sideways and supporting it with a pillow, if required. You can also place a folded blanket below the ankles if your partner requires lower-back support.

## Back Massage

You may wish to use a massage table or yoga mat with a soft blanket and soft towel placed beneath the area you intend to massage. Cover the parts of your partner's body that you will not be massaging with a blanket. Let your partner know that you will begin.

- Pour a teaspoonful of oil into the palm of your hands and rub your hands together to warm the oil.
- Begin at the lower end of the back with your whole hands moving in a clockwise movement, slowly moving up and around in the direction of the heart. Keep contact with the body and apply light pressure as you move up and encompass all the back muscles. Moving in these larger circular movements to cover the back in what is known as 'effleurage' movements. Ensure you do not place any pressure on the spine area throughout. Effleurage movements will evenly distribute the oil over the back and begin to relax the body.

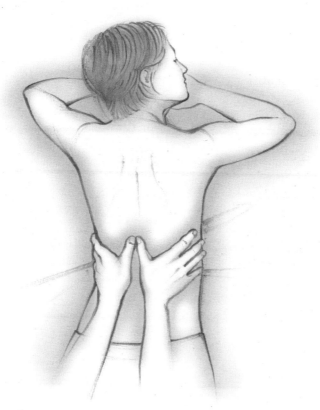

Back massage using effleurage movement

- Now begin again at the bottom of the back using 'petrissage' techniques. Your thumbs can move in a clockwise circular movement as you cover the lower back and sides of the body and then gently move up to cover all the back muscles. It is as though kneading bread with more of the rolling work being concentrated in the thumbs and directing the fingertips in smaller circular movements. The palms of the hand are raised off the body as the thumbs and fingertips roll and press gently across the back and shoulders for deeper relaxation.
- Begin this at the lower back, moving out to the waist and then slightly higher and in towards his/her core again, alternating between light to medium pressure. Keep your wrists relaxed throughout the back massage. Take between 10 and 15 minutes to massage the back and shoulder areas.
- As you move across the shoulder area, from the centre outwards, let your partner know that you are coming towards the end.

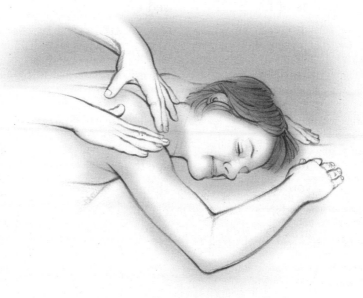

Back massage using petrissage movement

# CONCLUSION:

## *Bringing It All Together*

..................................................................................

A journey of a thousand miles begins with a single step.
LAO-TZU, CHINESE PHILOSOPHER (604–531 BC)

..................................................................................

By combining mind–body approaches with your fertility care, you are creating the optimum physical, emotional and psychological health to increase your chances of a successful pregnancy. Reading through this book you will have acquired clear and practical guidance in regards to assisted reproductive treatments, natural-healthcare approaches and evidence-based psychological and emotional support skills. This integrative healthcare approach is beneficial to your overall well-being and will keep you motivated to be true to your fertility goals with a balance of self-care and clear decision-making throughout.

When you embark on trying to conceive with fertility support, it can impact on many areas of your life. Following a review of the extensive research I have undertaken into the impact of fertility problems, I hope I have provided you with the essential resources to manage those areas that seem most affected by fertility issues, namely self-esteem, relationships, ways of thinking and emotions including feelings of grief, anger, stress and low mood. Identifying your own helpful and unhelpful beliefs and shining a spotlight on them with the help of CBT thought records will facilitate more balanced and supportive fertility thinking styles.

You also now have specific mindfulness practices you can use to help reduce stress and provide you with the insights and understanding you need to deal with any fertility challenges moving forward. Mindfulness exercises encourage deeper feelings of inner calm so that it is easier to manage any fluctuating feelings of joy and disappointment which often accompany the fertility process. With mindfulness, you are taught to be more aware of the moment-to-moment experience without being stuck in the fearful 'what ifs' of the past or the future. This has been proven to reduce stress and increase feelings of overall well-being. It allows you to connect to what is happening now and to make the best choices about what to do next in a responsive rather than reactive way. Evidence-based therapeutic skills, such as CBT and mindfulness, support you to manage challenges without losing a sense of yourself or being overwhelmed emotionally.

Whether you are new to fertility treatment or have already undertaken assisted reproductive care, understanding your medical treatment choices will prepare you to consider one medical approach over another and will also provide insight into what to expect from your treatment and your clinician. You now also understand how you can benefit from the curative power of expressive writing on an emotional and physiological level. Journaling throughout the fertility process helps you to reflect and be congruent to your hopes, desires and treatment choices. It will also help you to take space for some personal reflection when experiencing any loss or difficulties. Journaling regularly will ensure that you can gain the most from treatment and your consultations, and it will also provide you with the resources to cultivate self and relationship care throughout your treatment. In terms of relating successfully with medical and fertility care professionals, you now have the skills to gain the most from these interactions with assertiveness and open communication styles, ensuring that throughout your fertility journey you are most likely to express your needs and relate in optimal ways to secure the best outcomes.

It is so important when facing fertility problems to ensure that you and your partner are placed firmly in the centre of your fertility journey and that you have the tools to bring intimacy and closeness back into your relationship. By re-engaging with a deeper listening to each other and recognizing when you have become stuck in unhealthy relationship communication styles, you will be better able to express your needs in healthy and empathic ways and begin to bring the focus back into caring for the relationship and each other.

Bringing together fertility-specific health-promoting body and mind approaches, this book includes information on how to experience the health and healing available with natural health therapies in addition to conventional medical approaches. It also helps you to choose effective therapies and the most appropriate practitioners to meet your fertility needs. Offering clear and easy-to-follow nutritional advice, women's health specialist Dr Marilyn Glenville has shown you how to effectively support your fertility chances with dietary changes and fertility-specific supplements. Combining these changes with the health benefits of restorative yoga will ensure that your body feels strong, energized and balanced.

Planning to have a baby with natural or assisted fertility treatment draws on all your strengths and energy. You are now able to navigate your fertility journey in a self-empowered and proactive way, restoring harmony to your mind and body, and optimizing your chances of conception. You now also have the skills to successfully communicate your fertility needs, meaning you can be true to yourself and your relationship. The supportive, practical strategies outlined throughout the book will help you to make treatment choices with clarity and enable you to manage all aspects of your fertility process with less stress and more confidence. I hope that the step-by-step skills learned in this book will help you to be kind to yourself and experience equanimity throughout your fertility journey.

## Ten Steps to Mind–Body Balance

### Step 1: A Healthy Mind Promotes a Healthy Body

Understanding how repeated stress can impact on your body can help you to move out of automatic pilot and become more aware of the symptoms before they escalate. It is important to understand the difference between anxiety versus concern, and low mood versus sadness, and how to support yourself during challenging times. By understanding grief and loss you will be enabled to move through the healing process and, if necessary, choose a fertility-counselling approach suited to your needs.

### Step 2: Take Charge of your Mind–Body Fertility Health

Mindfulness increases our ability to recognize our stress triggers and respond rather than react to them. Increasing mindful awareness will help you to manage psychological, physiological and emotional fertility-related experiences in a calm and clear way. Incorporating mindfulness-based stress reduction for fertility skills, such as sitting meditations, the three-minute mindful check-in, the body scan, restorative yoga and mindful walking meditations, will enable you to feel empowered and deeply relaxed.

### Step 3: Utilize the Healing Power of Journaling

Keeping a journal is both therapeutic and pragmatic. It offers a non-judgemental space in which to express difficult or repeated thoughts and emotions. This will help you to reflect on and overcome any issues before moving forward with confidence. Journaling helps you to access your 'wise mind' – bringing balance to your emotional and reasoning self, important for any decision-making or healing process.

### Step 4: Understanding Your Medical Treatment Choices

I regularly hear individuals and couples express that they wish they'd known what was involved in their treatment options so that they could have considered the implications of one treatment choice over another. It is important to bear in mind the short- and long-term implications of each treatment choice and how to gain the most from it.

### Step 5: Use Natural Health Therapies to Enhance Your Conception Chances

Whether you choose acupuncture, aromatherapy, naturopathy or biodynamic massage, complementary therapies have been shown to promote your overall fertility health. Natural health therapy is key in supporting the physical process of fertility.

### Step 6: Use Nutrition and Supplements to Boost Fertility

Making certain diet and lifestyle choices, as well as taking supplements with fertility-boosting nutrients, supports your overall fertility health and can improve your natural conception chances, as well as complementing your assisted reproductive treatment.

### Step 7: Balance Your Body and Mind with Restorative Yoga and Mindful Movement

Restorative yoga and mindful movement can reduce physical tension and the physiological impact of treatment as well as restore self-compassion by focusing on reconnecting you with your body and regaining your intuitive wisdom.

### Step 8: Take a Solution-focused Approach to Your Mind Health

Cognitive behavioural therapy (CBT) is an evidence-based therapeutic approach that can help you to recognize and change any thoughts or beliefs that do not support you on your fertility journey. The skills gained by integrating CBT can work towards improving all areas of your life and relationships, by increasing positive change in how you think and what you do to improve how you feel.

## Step 9: Nurture Yourself and Communicate Your Needs Effectively

Taking care of your emotional well-being will provide you with the resources to move through your fertility issues with more ease and self-compassion. It is easy to get lost in the appointments, injections and planning involved in fertility treatment. It is therefore important to refocus on other areas of your life, nurturing your self-care. Learning helpful communication and assertiveness skills will also benefit you in all your relationships, as well as ensuring your voice is heard in the consulting room.

## Step 10: Enhance Your Relationship

We all respond differently to stressful situations. For some couples it brings them closer together as they gain a deeper empathy and understanding towards each other. For others, it creates a rupture in the relationship as hurt deepens into toxic resentment towards one another. By understanding our relationship blueprints, we can begin to foster healthier and more loving relationship styles. Incorporating nurturing and conflict-resolution exercises also contributes towards caring attitudes and behaviours in the relationship. Healing touch and mindfulness practice can encourage intimacy, ensuring that you remain best friends throughout the positive and more challenging times of fertility treatment.

# ABOUT THE AUTHOR

**Ann Bracken** (MA, GradDip, PGCert) is a Specialist Fertility Counsellor and Cognitive Behavioural Psychotherapist working in private practice in Dublin, Ireland and Kensington, London, with couples and individuals, and internationally with an online counselling service: www.fertilitycounsellingonline.com. She combines this with a part-time role as Senior Fertility Counsellor at the world-renowned Lister Fertility Clinic, which is part of The Lister Hospital, Chelsea. Ann is also a part-time lecturer in the Department of Psychology at Glyndŵr University, Wales, lecturing in Family Therapy and Cognitive Behavioural Psychotherapy (CBT). As a certified Fertility Mind-Body Programme trainer, Ann delivers weekend and evening work-shops throughout Ireland and the UK.

Ann has previously worked as a Cognitive Behavioural Psychotherapist and Mindfulness Trainer in national health settings (UK and Ireland) and managed the fertility counselling service in SIMS IVF, part of the Virtus Health group with 15 fertility clinics worldwide.

Ann has also worked as a researcher on many health and features programmes during her time in BBC, RTÉ and TV3

Television. She is a published author and feature writer on emotional and psychological health and well-being.

## Further Support

Ann works therapeutically with individuals and couples in private practice in Kensington (London) and Dublin city centre (Ireland).

Ann also runs online fertility counselling, a service to support individuals via Skype or with telephone or email counselling. Further details and bookings can be made at: www.fertilitycoun-sellingonline.com

To book an appointment in Kensington, London:
Tel: (+44) 07594 057541
Email: appointments@annbrackentherapy.com

To book an appointment in Dublin, Ireland:
Tel: (+353) 0 85 7414866
Email: appointments@annbrackentherapy.com

**The Fertility Mind–Body Programme**

Ann Bracken is a certified mindfulness teacher and mind-body programme trainer. She facilitates weekend Fertility Mind–Body Programme workshops in London (UK) and in Dublin and Wicklow (Ireland).

The Fertility Mind–Body Programme provides a supportive environment for couples and individuals going through the fertility treatment process to reduce stress and enhance their fertility health and well-being.

This co-facilitated weekend programme includes mindfulness-based stress reduction, CBT, nutritional therapy, restorative yoga, relationship support and emotional coping strategies using positive psychology. The small groups offer a confidential and comfortable environment for mutual support.

For more details and to book your place on the Fertility Mind–Body Programme Weekend Workshop, please log on to: www.fertilitycounsellingonline.com

# USEFUL RESOURCES

**Adoption UK**
Helpline: 0844 848 7900
www.adoptionuk.org

**The American Society for Reproductive Medicine (ASRM)**
1209 Montgomery Highway
Birmingham
Alabama 35216-2809
USA
Tel: (205) 978 5000
www.asrm.org

**British Infertility Counselling Association (BICA)**
www.bica.net

**The Daisy Network**
PO Box 71432
London SW6 9HJ
www.daisynetwork.org.uk

**Domar Center for Mind/Body Health**

130 Second Avenue

Waltham, MA 02451

USA

Tel: (781) 434 6578

www.domarcenter.com

**Donor Conception Network**

154 Caledonian Road

London N1 9RD

Tel. 020 7278 2608

www.dcnetwork.org

**Dr Marilyn Glenville**

14 St John's Road

Tunbridge Wells TN4 9NP

Tel: 08705 329 244

Int: +44 1892 515905

www.marilynglenville.com

**Emma Cannon's Fertility Rooms**

19 Cliveden Place

London SW1W 8HD

Tel: 07531 916121

www.emmacannon.co.uk

**European Society of Human Reproduction and Embryology
(ESHRE)**

Meerstraat 60

B-1852 Grimbergen

Belgium
Tel: +32 (0)2 269 09 69
www.eshre.eu

**Human Fertilisation & Embryology Authority (HFEA)**
Finsbury Tower
103–105 Bunhill Row
London EC1Y 8HF
Tel: 020 7291 8200
www.hfea.gov.uk

**The Infertility Network (UK)**
Charter House
43 St Leonards Road
Bexhill on Sea
East Sussex TN40 1JA
Helpline: 0800 008 7464
www.infertilitynetworkuk.com

**The Miscarriage Association**
17 Wentworth Terrace
Wakefield WF1 3QW
Helpline: 01924 200 799
www.miscarriageassociation.org.uk

# NOTES

CHAPTER 1 Managing the Psychological and Emotional
Impact of Fertility Problems

1 Boivin, J., et al. (2007). International estimates of infertility prevalence and treatment-seeking: potential need and demand for infertility medical care. *Human Reproduction*, 22(6), 1506–1512

2 European Society of Human Reproduction and Embryology (July 2014). Assistant Reproductive Treatment Fact Sheet, www.eshre. eu/guidelines-and-legal/ART-fact-sheet (accessed: 03.09.15)

3 Bracken, A. (2013). Infertility and mental health: an analysis of Irish patient needs and evaluation of mindfulness-based cognitive therapy as a treatment model. Master's thesis, ICHAS and Sims IVF (part of Virtus Health Group)

4 Boivin, J., Takefman, J., Braverman, A. (2011). The fertility quality of life (FertiQoL) tool: development and general psychometric properties. *Human Reproduction*, 26(8), 2084–2091

5 Ibid.

6 Joy J. (2015). Consultant Gynaecologist and Subspecialist in Reproductive Medicine for *The Obstetrician & Gynaecologist (TOG)*, The Royal College of Obstetricians and Gynaecologists

7 Ibid.

8 Golombok, S., et al. (2011). Children conceived by gamete donation: psychological adjustment and mother-child relationships at age 7. *Journal of Family Psychology*, 25(2), 230–239

9 Berga, S., Loucks, T. (2006). Use of cognitive behavior therapy for functional hypothalamic amenorrhea. *Annals of the New York Academy of Sciences*, 1092(1), 114–129

10 Olivius, C., Fridén, B., Borg, G., Bergh, C. (2002). Psychological aspects of discontinuation of in vitro fertilization treatment. *Fertility and Sterility*, 81(2), 276

11 Kübler-Ross, E. (1969). *On Death and Dying*. New York: Macmillan

CHAPTER 2 Mindfulness Practice

1 Kabat-Zinn, J. (2005). *Wherever You Go, There You Are*. New York: Hyperion

2 Pickert, K. (2014). The mindful revolution: finding focus in a stressed-out and multitasking culture. *Time Magazine*, *3 February*, 34–38

3 Kabat-Zinn, J. (1990). *Full Catastrophe Living*. London: Piatkus

4 Domar, A. D., et al. (2011). Impact of a group mind/body intervention on pregnancy rates in IVF patients. *Fertility and Sterility*, 95(7), 2269–2273

5 Prince L. B., Domar A. (2011). Impact of psychological interventions on IVF outcome. *SRM Journal of Mediscience*, 9, 26–32

6 Hammerli, K., Znoj, H., Barth, J. (2009). The efficacy of psychological interventions for infertile patients; a meta-analysis examining mental health and pregnancy rate. *Human Reproduction* 15(3), 279–295

7 Boivin, J., et al. (2011). Emotional distress in infertile women

and failure of assisted reproductive technologies: meta-analysis of prospective psychosocial studies. *BMJ*, 342

8 Nakamura, K., et al. (2008). Stress and reproductive failure: past notions, present insights and future directions. *Journal of Assisted Reproduction and Genetics*, 25(2–3), 47–62

9 Lynch, C. D., et al. (2014). Preconception stress increases the risk of infertility: results from a couple-based prospective cohort study – the LIFE study. *ESHRE Journal. Human Reproduction*, 29(5), 1067–1075

10 Louis, G., et al. (2011). Stress reduces conception probabilities across the fertile window: evidence in support of relaxation. *Fertility and Sterility*, 95(7), 2184–2189

11 Boyles, S. (2010). Stress may affect chances of getting pregnant, http://www.webmd.com/baby/news/20100812/stress-may-affect-chances-of-getting-pregnant (accessed: 05.09.2015)

12 Glenville, M. (2012). *Getting Pregnant Faster*. London: Kyle Books

13 Pennebaker, J. (2004). *Writing to Heal*. Oakland, CA: New Harbinger

14 Benson, H. (2000). *The Relaxation Response*. NY: HarperCollins

15 Scherer, M. (2012). 2012 Person of the Year: Barack Obama, the President. *Time Magazine*, December 2012/January 2013, http://poy.time.com/2012/12/19/times-person-of-the-year-issue-cover-gallery/slide/person-of-the-year-president-barack-obama/ (accessed: 20.09.15)

16 Monteith, S. (2008). *American Culture in the 1960s*. Edinburgh: Edinburgh University Press, 129

17 Baikie, K., Wilhelm, K. (2005). Emotional and physical health benefits of expressive writing. *Advances in Psychiatric Treatment*, 11(5), 338–346

18 Pennebaker, J., et al. (1988), Esterling, B. A., et al. (1994), Booth, R. J., et al. (1997), Baikie, K., et al. (2005). In: Baikie, K., Wilhelm, K. (2005). Emotional and physical health benefits of expressive writing. *Advances in Psychiatric Treatment*, 11(5), 338–346

19 Baikie, K., Wilhelm, K. (2005). Emotional and physical health benefits of expressive writing. *Advances in Psychiatric Treatment*, 11(5), 338–346

20 Domar, A. D., Zuttermeister, P. C., Friedman, R. (1993). The psychological impact of infertility: a comparison with patients with other medical conditions. *Journal of Psychosomatic Obstetrics and Gynaecology*, 14, 45–52

## CHAPTER 3  Assisted Reproductive Treatment

1 National Institute for Health and Care Excellence (NICE) (2013). Fertility: Assessment and treatment for people with fertility problems. Guideline CG156

2 Ibid.

3 Ibid.

4 Human Fertilisation & Embryology Authority (HFEA) (2015). Facts and Figures, Latest UK IVF figures: 2010 and 2011, http://www.hfea.gov.uk/ivf-figures-2006.html#1276 (accessed: 09.15)

5 Balázs, K. (2010/12). A kései gyermekvállalás kockázatai. *KorFa on-line*, http://www.demografia.hu/kiadvanyokonline/index.php/korfa/article/view/791/246 (accessed 26.08.2012)

6 Olivius, C. (2009). *Cumulative Live Birth Rates after In Vitro Fertilization*. Gothenburg: University of Gothenburg

7 Sherbahn, R. (2013). High AMH Levels in Women Under Age 35 Undergoing IVF Are Correlated With High Live Birth Rates. Women With Very Low AMH Levels Have High Cancellation Rates but Reasonable Live Birth Rates. Research study presented

at the 69th Annual Meeting of the American Society for Reproductive Medicine, Boston, MA

8 Borrero, C. (2001). Gamete and embryo donation. In: *Current practices and controversies in assisted reproduction.* Report of a meeting on medical, ethical and social aspects of assisted reproduction. Geneva: World Health Organization

9 Ockhuijsen, H., et al. (2013). The PRCI study: design of a randomized clinical trial to evaluate a coping intervention for medical waiting periods used by women undergoing a fertility treatment. *BMC women's health*, 13(1), 35

CHAPTER 4 Natural Health Therapies

1 World Health Organization (2002). Acupuncture: review and analysis of reports on controlled clinical trials

2 Paulus, W. E., et al. (2002). Influence of acupuncture on the pregnancy rate in patients who undergo assisted reproduction therapy. *Fertility and Sterility*, 77(4), 721–724

3 Smith, C., Coyle, M., Norman, R. J. (2006). Influence of acupuncture stimulation on pregnancy rates for women undergoing embryo transfer. *Fertility and Sterility*, 85(5), 1352–1358

4 Longbottom, J. (2008). The use of acupuncture with in vitro fertilization: is there a point? *Journal of the Association of Chartered Physiotherapists in Women's Health*, 103, 29–38

5 Manheimer, E., et al. (2008). Effects of acupuncture on rates of pregnancy and live birth among women undergoing in vitro fertilisation: systematic review and meta-analysis. *BMJ*, 336(7643), 545–549

6 Gray, M. (2008). Health News, NHS Choices. http://www.nhs.uk/news/2007/January08/Pages/AcupunctureandsuccessofIVF.aspx (accessed 09.2015)

7  Zhang, J., et al. (2010). Acupuncture-related adverse events: a systematic review of the Chinese literature. *Bulletin of the World Health Organization*, 88(12), 915–921

8  Gattefossé, R. M. (1937). *Aromathérapie: les huiles essentielles hormones végétales*, Paris: Girardot

9  Schaible, M. (2008). Biodynamic massage as a body therapy, and as a tool in body therapy. In: Hartley, L. (2008). *Contemporary body psychotherapy: the Chiron approach* Hove: Routledge, 31–35

CHAPTER 5 Using Nutrition and Supplements to Boost Fertility by Dr Marilyn Glenville

1  Office for National Statistics (2014). Live Births in England and Wales by Characteristics of Mother 1, 2013

2  Harris, I. D., et al. (2011). Fertility and the Aging Male. *Reviews in Urology*, 13(4), e184–e190

3  Human Fertilisation & Embryology Authority (HFEA). Fertility Treatment in 2011: Trends and Figures, http://www.hfea.gov.uk /docs/HFEA_Fertility_Trends_and_Figures_2011_-_Annual_ Register_Report.pdf

4  Marsh, K. A., et al. (2010). Effect of a low glycemic index compared with a conventional healthy diet on polycystic ovary syndrome. *The American Journal of Clinical Nutrition*, 92, 83–92

5  Chavarro, J. E., et al. (2008). Protein intake and ovulatory infertility. *American Journal of Obstetrics & Gynecology*, 198(2), 210e1–210e7

6  Lintsen, B. (2008). Presented at the European Society of Human Reproduction and Embryology's annual conference

7  Weng, X., et al. (2008). Maternal caffeine consumption during pregnancy and the risk of miscarriage: a prospective cohort

study. *American Journal of Obstetrics and Gynecology*, 198(3), 279e1–279e8

8  Nawrt, P., et al. (2003). Effects of caffeine on human health. *Food Additives & Contaminants*, 20(1), 1–30

9  Tolstrup, J. S., et al. (2003). Alcohol use as predictor for infertility in a representative population of Danish women. *Acta Obstetricia et Gynecologica Scandinavica*, 82(8), 744–749

10  Guo, H., et al. (2006). Effects of cigarette, alcohol consumption and sauna on sperm morphology. *Zhonghua Nan Ke Xue*, 12(3), 215–217

11  ASH. Smoking and Reproduction. Research studies fact sheet, 2000

12  BMA report, 2004

13  Guo, H., et al. (2006). Effects of cigarette, alcohol consumption and sauna on sperm morphology. *Zhonghua Nan Ke Xue*, 12(3), 215–217

14  Klonoff-Cohen, H., et al. (2001). Effects of female and male smoking on success rates of IVF and gamete intra-fallopian transfer. *Human Reproduction*, 16(7), 1382–1390

15  Sheynkin, Y., et al. (2005). Increase in scrotal temperature in laptop computer users. *Human Reproduction*, 20(2), 452–455

16  Hassan, M., et al. (2004). Negative lifestyle is associated with a significant reduction in fecundity. *Fertility and Sterility*, 81(2), 384–392

17  Wong, W. Y., et al. (2002). Effects of folic acid and zinc sulfate on male factor subfertility: a double-blind randomized, placebo-controlled trial. *Fertility and Sterility*, 77(3), 491–498

18  Safarinejad, M. R., Safarinejad, S. (2009). Efficacy of selenium and/or N-acetyl-cysteine for improving semen parameters in infertile men: a double-blind, placebo controlled, randomized study. *The Journal of Urology*, 181(2), 741–751

19 Greco, E., et al. (2005). ICSI in cases of sperm DNA damage: beneficial effect of oral antioxidant treatment. *Human Reproduction*, 20(9), 2590–2594

20 Tarin, J., et al. (1998). Effects of maternal ageing and dietary antioxidant supplementation on ovulation, fertilisation and embryo development in vitro in the mouse. *Reproduction Nutrition Development*, 38(5), 499–508

21 Ruder, E. H., et al. (2014). Female dietary antioxidant intake and time to pregnancy among couples treated for unexplained infertility. *Fertility and Sterility*, 101(3), 759–66

22 Showell, M. G., et al. (2011). Antioxidants for male subfertility. *Cochrane Database of Systematic Reviews*, Jan 19(1), CD007411

23 Srivastava, S. (2006). Mechanism of action of l-arginine on the vitality of spermatozoa is primarily through increased biosynthesis of nitric oxide. *Biology of Reproduction*, 74(5), 954–958

24 Gurbuz, B., et al. (2003). Relationship between semen quality and seminal plasma total carnitine in infertile men. *Journal of Obstetrics and Gynecology*, 23(6), 653–656

25 Rossi, E., et al. (1993). Fish oil derivatives as a prophylaxis of recurrent miscarriage associated with antiphospholipid antibodies (APL): a pilot study. *Lupus*, 2(5), 319–323

26 Safarinejad, M. R. (2011). Effect of omega-3 polyunsaturated fatty acid supplementation on semen profile and enzymatic antioxidant capacity of seminal plasma in infertile men with idiopathic oligoasthenoteratospermia: a double-blind, placebo-controlled, randomised study. *Andrologia*, 43(1), 38–47

27 Hayes, C. E., et al. (2003). The immunological functions of the vitamin D endocrine system. *Cellular and Molecular Biology*, 49(2), 277–300

28 Panda, D. K., et al. (2001). Targeted ablation of the 25-hydrox-yvitamin D 1alpha-hydroxylase enzyme: evidence for skeletal, reproductive, and immune dysfunction. *Proceedings of the National Academy of Sciences*, 98(13), 7498–7503

29 Jensen, M. B., et al. (2011). Vitamin D is positively associated with sperm motility and increases intracellular calcium in human spermatozoa. *Human Reproduction*, 26(6), 1307–1317

30 Pearce, S. H., Cheetham, T.D. (2010). Diagnosis and manage-ment of vitamin D deficiency. *BMJ*, 340(7738), 142–147

31 Safarinejad, M. R. (2009). Efficacy of coenzyme Q10 on semen parameters, sperm function and reproductive hormones in infertile men. *The Journal of Urology*, 182(1), 237–248

32 Bentov, Y., Casper, R. (2013). The aging oocyte – can mitochon-drial function be improved? *Fertility and Sterility*, 99(1), 18–22

33 Ben-Meir, A., et al. (2015). Coenzyme Q10 restores oocyte mitochondrial function and fertility during reproductive aging. *Aging Cell*, 14(5), 887–895

34 Comhaire, F. (2010). The role of food supplementation in the treatment of the infertile couple and for assisted reproduction. *Andrologia*, 42(5), 331–340

CHAPTER 6 Restorative Yoga and Mindful Movement

1 Jacobson, E. (1938). *Progressive Relaxation*. Chicago: University of Chicago Press

CHAPTER 9 Caring for Your Relationship and Understanding Each Other

1 Brach, T. (2013). *True Refuge*. UK: Hayhouse

2 Post, S. (2011). *The Hidden Gifts of Helping: How the power of giving, compassion and hope can get us through hard times*. CA: Jossey-Bass

# INDEX

Note Page numbers in **bold** refer to diagrams.

## yellow kite

books to help you live a good life

Join the conversation and tell
us how you live a #goodlife

@yellowkitebooks
YellowKiteBooks
Yellow Kite Books
YellowKiteBooks